Nature's Secret Messages

Hay House Titles of Related Interest

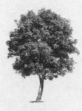

Praise for *Nature's Secret Messages*

"This wise, brave, magically simple, and inspiring book will help us all reconnect with the soul of nature, and work together to preserve the environment and the human adventure."

— **Andrew Harvey,** the *New York Times* best-selling author of *The Hope: A Guide to Sacred Activism*

"A wonderful book with pearls of wisdom on every page."

— **Stephen Harrod Buhner,** ecologist, and the author of the multiple award-winning book *The Lost Language of Plants*

"Fascinating book! Thank you, Elaine, for bringing Nature's secrets back to life and reuniting mankind with the earth."

— **Laurentine ten Bosch,** the co-producer of *Food Matters*

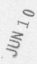

Nature's Secret Messages

hidden in plain sight

Elaine Wilkes

HAY HOUSE, INC.

Carlsbad, California • New York City
London • Sydney • Johannesburg
Vancouver • Hong Kong • New Delhi

Published and distributed in the United States by: Hay House, Inc.: www.hay house.com • *Published and distributed in Australia by:* Hay House Australia Pty. Ltd.: www.hayhouse.com.au • *Published and distributed in the United Kingdom by:* Hay House UK, Ltd.: www.hayhouse.co.uk • *Published and distributed in the Republic of South Africa by:* Hay House SA (Pty), Ltd.: www.hayhouse.co.za • *Distributed in Canada by:* Raincoast: www.raincoast.com • *Published in India by:* Hay House Publishers India: www.hayhouse.co.in

Editorial supervision: Jill Kramer • *Design:* Julie Davison

Front-cover photos: **iStockphoto.com** (walnut and brain); **Dreamstime.com** (tree)

The photos on the following pages are from **iStockphoto.com**: 7 (left), 12, 17 (left), 25, 28, 29, 37, 50, 60, 63 (right), 65, 67, 96, 111, 118, 129 (first, third, fifth), 130, 133 (all left side, middle right), 134, 140, 143 (left), 144 (bottom right).
The photos on the following pages are from **Dreamstime.com**: 7 (right), 17 (right), 21, 30, 35, 36, 38, 40, 48 (left), 63 (left), 69 (right), 79, 87, 129 (second, fourth, sixth), 133 (top right), 136, 137, 138, 143 (right), 144 (all left side).
The photos on pages 122, 221, and 223 are courtesy of the author.

Library of Congress Cataloging-in-Publication Data

Wilkes, Elaine.
  Nature's secret messages : hidden in plain sight / Elaine Wilkes. -- 1st ed.
    p. cm.
  ISBN 978-1-4019-2546-8 (tradepaper : alk. paper) 1. Nature, Healing power of. 2. Self-care, Health. 3. Mind and body. I. Title.
  R723.W545 2010
  615.5--dc22

                                            2009026064

ISBN: 978-1-4019-2546-8

13 12 11 10   4 3 2 1
1st edition, February 2010

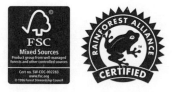

Printed in the United States of America

*For my Mom, Ruth ("Rootie"), who
was there wholeheartedly through every step
of this book; and whose wisdom, inspiring insights,
editing, fact-checking assistance, enthusiasm,
and love are poured over all of these pages.*

Contents

PART III: Nature's Secrets about Our Spiritual Journey

**PART IV: Nature's Secrets about Food, Drugs,
and Deception**

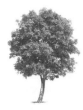

PREFACE

How This Book Came to Be

"Hello, my name is Elaine."

"Welcome, Elaine."

"I'm a learning addict."

Some people turn to booze, gambling, or drugs. Throughout my life, I turned to classes, seminars, and books on health, growth, and empowerment. No, you wouldn't find me at the local bar or sleazy gin joint—instead, I was hanging out, bleary-eyed, at the local library until closing time, wanting "one more book for the road."

My learning addiction started when I was about 14 years old. My dad, who grew up dirt poor and became a self-made man, got me hooked on his countless tapes on positive thinking, visualization, and success principles. As a teenager, I put his advice to the test: I visualized myself winning a contest for *Teen* magazine, being chosen from thousands of entrants and celebrating the prize of an all-expenses-paid weeklong trip to California. Living in the Midwest, I saw this as an exotic, dreamy adventure.

The visualization tapes instructed me to imagine every detail of the scenario, so I made it into a game. First thing in the morning and before I went to sleep at night, I visualized myself winning the contest. It didn't take much effort to do this; it was actually fun to imagine more details to add to my picture. I even marked the dates in my calendar when I'd be vacationing in California.

When I got the official call informing me that I'd actually won the contest, I was excited but not all that surprised . . . I felt more like, *Oh yeah, I'm ready for it!*

For years, I played similar "imagination games." I guess I still do, because in this book I talk about how to view Nature and life in fresh, imaginative ways. I've developed a "habit" for mainlining Norman Vincent Peale, Wayne Dyer, and Napoleon Hill—each one of these wise teachers taught me to create by painting pictures on the canvas of my mind. For instance, I painted myself as an actress, which eventually resulted in an exclusive contract with NBC, followed by roles in numerous movies and TV shows with A-list actors, including Madonna, Bruce Willis, Courteney Cox, Larry Hagman, Mark Harmon, Kim Basinger, and Kate Capshaw. I also appeared in more than 75 commercials.

I then went for a new high, which fed my learning addiction even further. In order to stretch my mind and abilities, I started a business creating presentations on health, mind, body, and soul for corporations and speakers such as Deepak Chopra, M.D., and Barry Sears, Ph.D. (the author of *The Zone*). Over the years, I've developed and attended hundreds of presentations, absorbing countless gems of wisdom that now enrich this book.

Then I got sick. *Really* sick. A nutritionist gave me vitamins made by a small, unknown company, which had processed the ingredients incorrectly, causing me to ingest highly toxic levels of minerals. I became so ill that I lost all of my hair and fingernails, and my upper body was covered in rashes. I learned firsthand that poor health is the gutter of all lows. *Norman Vincent Peale, where are you?!*

I also experienced the incredible power of words. Before I lost my hair, I often complained, "Oh, I hate my hair!" But when I was sick and it started falling out in clumps, I cried, "Nooo! I love my hair!" Too late, unfortunately. Now I'm grateful that my hair grew back, and that I *have* hair. I've come to believe that one's soul is deeply injured by those types of loathing, glib remarks.

During this dark time in my life, I realized that battling a disease or illness has a way of consuming all energy and thoughts, leaving sufferers gripped by fear. I often found myself wondering,

Will I ever get better? Is this a permanent way of life? When life is engulfed in a gloomy fog, how do we find our way out?

For me, my illness was a bottoming-out experience. Now I'm amazed when I see people treating their cars better than they treat themselves. They think nothing of spending money on premium fuel for their engine, but skimp on their own body, choosing low-quality "fuel" and ignoring the ways in which it influences their health, weight, energy, mood, and mental ability. Our bodies drive our lives—we must do whatever we can to keep them running smoothly.

My illness also fueled my learning addiction. I grew passionate about restoring my health, which led me to complete a master's degree in psychology, become a nutritionist, earn a Ph.D. in naturopathy (healing through natural methods), and even earn a certification as a Kundalini yoga/meditation instructor.

I began to discover Nature's profound secrets and ancient mysteries while writing my Ph.D. dissertation. As I pored over countless studies and texts from ancient through modern times, and as I interviewed scientists, researchers, farmers, healers, shamans, ethnobotanists, and herbalists from all over the world, this "information-oholic" was on a tremendous high.

I found Nature to be the most fascinating, inspiring, and charismatic teacher I'd ever encountered. And by relying on Mother Nature as my guide, I began to assemble all of my knowledge (a smorgasbord of Zen, Christian, Taoist, Kabbalistic, Chinese, Ayurvedic, American, Native American, shamanic, and botanical wisdom, as well as various other teachings and traditions) on even deeper levels. This freed me from my information addiction. Today, I access my inner guidance and consult with Nature one day at a time.

What I've Gathered from This Intensive Learning, and How It Can Help You

I propose that Nature is more profound than anyone can imagine and is always giving you signs. Learning Nature's "language" can be life changing. Nature is your most vital teacher, the one you've been waiting for.

This book presents Nature's prescription for better health and a deeper connection to yourself and the planet. You'll reconnect with the wonder and imagination you felt as a child, helping you to see yourself, the earth, and the food you eat in a whole new light. It's a one-way ticket to a fresh, exciting way to create positive inner and outer changes.

For me, tuning in to Nature's intelligence was like when Dorothy entered the magical Land of Oz: everything suddenly changed from black and white to Technicolor. My eyes opened to the marvels of colors and shapes all around me. I noticed things that I never had before and discovered newfound comfort in the natural world. In the past, I'd been very similar to Dorothy, who had been wearing the ruby slippers the entire time but didn't know that they had the power to take her home. *I* had the magic within reach, but I had to discover how to access it. Like Dorothy's slippers, Nature's wisdom can go unnoticed in today's busy, technologically intensive world.

Try imagining a well-worn trail on the ground, and alongside it, grass that could become a trail, too, if walked on many times. You've been traveling the same worn path over and over, but what if, instead, you started forging a different route through the grass? All you have to do is choose to move in a new direction.

Now is the time for a magical voyage into Nature. Prepare to experience the world, and yourself, in fresh, wondrous ways. And if questions come up on this unfamiliar journey, which they will, all you need to do is simply ask, "What would Nature do?"

My sincere wish is that Nature becomes your true friend and mentor, and that this book fills you with many "awe-ha" moments. Let Mother Nature's show-and-tell begin!

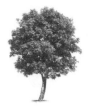

INTRODUCTION

*"Come forth into the light of things,
Let nature be your teacher."*

— **William Wordsworth**

Einstein once said, "Look deep into nature, and then you will understand everything better." What he was getting at is that Mother Nature is our role model.

In today's "modern" society, we too often forget to look to Nature—with her four billion years of knowledge and experience—as our mentor and nurturer. Yet when we do remember, we find that she holds the answers, offering us an abundance of cures for our ailments; nourishment for our bodies; and prescriptions for achieving physical, emotional, and spiritual health. Our most profound and inspirational teacher, our greatest role model, is right outside our front door . . . and her lifelong lessons are free! It's time for us to reconnect to this relationship and discover Nature's secret messages so that we can use this ancient, intuitive wisdom to heal the planet and ourselves.

How This Book Is Set Up

Part I: Nature's Secrets about Appearances and Physical Health details how Nature gives clues through a plant's appearance on how it might be able to improve your physical health. To be able to decode those secrets, however, you must first be willing to use your intuition and imagination, so this section of the book also outlines how you can learn to open up to that part of your inner wisdom and curiosity.

Remember when you were a child and saw possibilities everywhere? An old broom could suddenly become a witch's flying broomstick, a pony, or a magic wand! In general, kids have more fun than adults because they access their *nonthinking* imagination— that is, they explore the world with wonder. Busy adults usually see that broom as something that only sweeps up dirt.

Get ready to stretch your right-brained creativity *and* your left-brained rational thinking skills, as you'll also delve into plenty of science and research that backs up the information presented. Even if you end up looking at this part of the book as merely a collection of innovative ways to remember facts about foods and plants, it will undoubtedly *plant* a seed in your mind that will eventually grow into an increased awareness of the mysteries in Nature.

Part II: Nature's Secrets about Emotional and Mental Well-Being looks at how Nature's symbolism can guide you in managing your emotions. In this section, you'll learn how to avoid the pressure of time by recognizing Mother Nature's rhythms and using them as a powerful model. You'll also learn to successfully navigate change—a vital skill in today's fast-paced world. Why do certain species in Nature not only welcome change and survive, but also thrive in the midst of turmoil? In what ways do some creatures work together, sharing intelligence to serve the larger group and ensuring everyone's survival? You'll read all about that here.

At the end of Part II, you'll take Nature's wisdom on a trip to Las Vegas and learn her winning formulas. If you've never thought of yourself as being particularly lucky before, get ready to change all that! Luck, it turns out, is hardly random—it's a quality you can acquire . . . if you know how to tap into Nature's secret messages.

Part III: Nature's Secrets about Our Spiritual Journey shows how seemingly haphazard events in Nature may indeed have a vital purpose. After all, Nature isn't always a bed of roses! Observing how this bigger picture works in the natural world can help you understand how unexpected events in your own life may not be so coincidental.

You'll also read about Mother Nature's patterns and how they can mirror the patterns of *your* inner nature, illustrating how you are indeed intertwined with everyone else on the planet, as well as with all creation. Recognizing this interconnection can help you develop a deep intimacy with the natural world that will lead to a richly fulfilling and peaceful life, in balance with all that is.

Part IV: Nature's Secrets about Food, Drugs, and Deception deals with the importance of being in harmony with Earth, particularly in the ways in which food is grown and marketed. You'll read about what happens to your food along the way from the farmer's field to store shelves and what it's costing you. You may think that you're being a smart shopper picking the prettiest produce, but you're about to discover the ugly truth. In fact, you may totally reevaluate the way you shop for food and what you buy! This final part also explores small steps you can take to make a huge difference in helping to heal the planet.

Sprinkled throughout the book are numerous insightful "Nature's Secrets," as well as quick "Test Your Nature IQ" quizzes just for fun.

Prepare to marvel as you learn natural ways to tune in to your own wisdom and reconnect to the natural world. Your "mother" really does know best! The more you know about Nature and heed her profound advice, the more you'll understand yourself and others.

I hope that *Nature's Secret Messages* will become a springboard for endless wonder, vision, and nurturing in your life . . . compliments of Nature.

🌿 🌿 🌿　 🌿 🌿 🌿

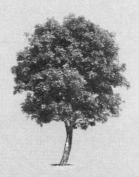

Part 1

Nature's Secrets about
Appearances and Physical Health

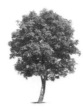

CHAPTER ONE

Stop, Look, Listen

"We lie in the lap of immense intelligence."

— **Ralph Waldo Emerson**

Stop. Look. Listen. My kindergarten teacher taught me that. I remember carefully lining up the tips of my patent-leather shoes exactly at the edge of the curb and stopping—then carefully looking to my right and left, quiet and aware, listening for any clues. Feeling that it was safe to proceed, I'd grasp my classmate's hand, jump off the curb, and happily venture into unknown territories on the other side of the street.

Now I barely glance from side to side as I hurry on my way.

What happened? Where did that wide-open feeling of awareness go? In the rush of adulthood, it seems to vanish, but what would happen if we simply stopped, looked, and listened . . . even as busy adults?

As a learning addict, I've hunted for insights through countless books, seminars, experts, masters, and more. Eventually, I realized that my kindergarten teacher had it right from the beginning, long before I started my quest. Who knew that she was so profound?

Stop, look, and listen to what's all around you, and all that's within you. *That's it.* That's the secret. Do just that and you'll positively change your life, for awareness opens the door to Nature's secrets—and they're *everywhere*.

Elementary Lessons

When I was a kindergartener perched on the sidewalk curb, I wasn't rushing. I wasn't thinking about whether or not I liked the "stop, look, and listen" rule, what I would be eating at lunchtime, or what my mother had said to me the night before. I was simply *aware* and in the moment, *feeling* that it was safe to move with joy. This is the experience of openness and observation.

People living in ancient civilizations also stopped, looked, and listened. In fact, they relied on these actions to survive. By observing what animals ate (and what they avoided), they found nourishment. However, this was only one method of learning about food and the healing potential of different plants. They also sought answers from shamans or spiritual leaders, who would commune with the plants' spirits.

Of course, trial and error was a reliable source of information as well. But with countless plants in the world—each with its own specific medicinal qualities and variation of leaves, roots, flowers, and fruits—the ancients were on the hunt for clues that might reveal something about the plant.

Just as a person's clothes and mannerisms can communicate messages to us, Nature communicates through her appearances. Through observation, reflection, intuition, and imagination, ancient people investigated the secret signs they believed the Creator provided about the power of each plant. For example, when they saw that the walnut looked like a brain (they most likely viewed this organ from the bodies of the animals they hunted and consumed), they interpreted it as a sign that walnuts were somehow beneficial for the functioning of their own brains.

"Plant wisdom" and other secrets of Nature have been handed down through generations. Hundreds of years ago, children could recite the names and traits of the natural life around them; their "celebrities" were plants and stars. If they'd had tabloids, they might have resembled our farmers' almanacs, filled with the latest "dirt" on which bees were pollinating which flowers! They didn't have the Internet, TVs, MP3 players, movies, radios, malls, cell phones, and other distractions . . . but they did use their blackberries (the edible ones)!

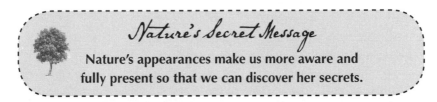

Nature's Secret Message

Nature's appearances make us more aware and fully present so that we can discover her secrets.

I've often wondered about the following: Are Nature's plans haphazard or methodical? Did the Creator give us clues to follow? If food is medicine, could these clues be Nature's prescriptions? Does our own food contain little mysteries?

Intrigued by these ideas, I started investigating and asked a scientist if the external characteristics of plants offered us any clues to their health benefits. As if dumping a bucket of cold water on me, the scientist shouted, "That's bull----! It's *not* science!" I posed the same question to a doctor, who condescendingly remarked, "You don't actually believe that, do you?" Along the same lines, a researcher replied, "Uh, nature isn't that cute." I mentioned the concept to a few male friends and heard lots of jokes about how men should eat large cucumbers more often.

I understood where they were all coming from, but considering Nature's incredible complexity, something inside of me kept pushing, *Why couldn't Mother Nature be throwing us a few clues?*

So I kept asking. By speaking with people who work with plants—including herbalists, farmers, and medicine women and men—I heard an entirely different story, one marked by honor, respect, and love of Nature's wonders.

Herbalist Matthew Wood became interested in Nature when he was 12 years old. On a school field trip, he recalled his teacher reciting: "Nature is alive, nature is alive! We live amid a living being."

Enlightened by that particular experience, Matthew went on to devote his life to studying Nature and her signs. When I asked him why so many people don't believe that plants, trees, and foods may have messages for us, he responded that the signs in Nature may not contain meaning until we can clearly observe and learn to read them. Unless someone spends time in Nature every day and has put in hundreds of working hours, he or she really can't understand just how much wisdom Nature provides.[1]

Another example, written in Malcolm Gladwell's book *Blink,* is when the Getty Museum purchased a statue for almost ten million dollars after conducting 14 months of exhaustive scientific tests to determine the relic's worth. However, an expert on Greek sculpture knew the second the statue was unveiled that something was off. And an art historian's initial impression was that the fingernails didn't look right. When viewing the statue, the first word that came to the director of the Metropolitan Museum of Art in New York was *fresh,* which is *not* a word associated with an ancient relic. After these instinctual gut feelings, it's no wonder that later it was discovered to be a fraud. These examples prove the point that when we're working on something day in, day out, our knowing can supersede scientific fact.

This reminded me of mothers who know precisely what their babies want from just a gurgle, gesture, or mumble, when everyone else perceives it as indiscernible baby talk or random movements. And, of course, when someone speaks in a language we don't understand, it doesn't mean they aren't communicating. If we can't read an illegible signature on a check, does that mean it's void? Not at all. It's the same with Nature's signs and clues: they may not hold any meaning for us until we learn to decipher them.

We can also see this phenomenon by examining ancient indigenous cultures throughout the world. Many of these people used plants in similar or identical ways, discovering Nature's secrets on their own, without communicating with each other. They've been able to do this by listening to their instincts and observing that the outer characteristics of plants often reveal their inner qualities. Our brilliant Creator hid these fabulous secrets in plain sight.

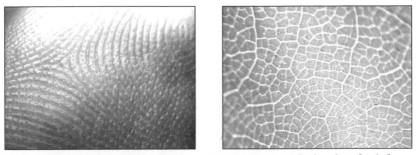

Fingerprints reveal so much about us. Can the "imprint" of a plant [right] also show us that there's a lot more going on below the surface?

How many times today did you notice genius around you? Okay, how many times this month or this year? Genius is *everywhere!*

Writer Gene Weingarten published a story in *The Washington Post* about a man who played the violin at a D.C. metro station during the morning rush hour. In 45 minutes, 1,097 people passed by, and only 7 stopped to listen. Twenty-seven of them gave him money, totaling $32, but most tossed the cash in his case as they rushed by. One child did stop, but his mother used her body to block the musician from sight so the child wouldn't become interested and linger.

What the commuters didn't realize was that this was an experiment and that Joshua Bell, one of the finest classical musicians in the world, was performing in their midst—*hidden in plain sight*. He was playing masterpieces that have been cherished for centuries on a $3.5 million violin. Only two days earlier, this award-winning musician had played for a sold-out audience who had paid a minimum ticket price of $100.[2]

According to the article, Joshua commented afterward that he'd felt invisible. When passersby were later asked about the performance in the station, one person who had been only four feet away asked, "Where was he?" Many preoccupied commuters who had hurriedly walked by reported that they missed seeing or hearing this musical genius altogether. Where were these people? Lost in their thoughts, that's where.

This experiment is a great analogy for most people's relationship with Nature. You have an orchestra playing around you every day, but it's invisible, hidden away, because you haven't stopped to notice Nature's genius. What treasures and magical opportunities are you passing by because of your business?

People who have observed Nature's signs have made numerous key discoveries. The humble scientist and inventor George Washington Carver attributed his understanding of crop rotation and ideas for using peanuts in hundreds of products to his love of observing Nature. Legendary herbalist Tommie Bass (who was honored with a *Wall Street Journal* cover-page tribute when he died) was so attuned to Nature's signs that he knew which plants would heal the thousands of people who sought help at his simple home in the mountains. This remarkable herbalist never attended a single day of school, except when he was invited to lecture on Nature's healing remedies at leading universities.

Nature's Works of Art

Like any great work of art, Nature's masterpieces are open to interpretation. Differing viewpoints can be equally valid. History professor William Eamon echoes this idea in his book *Science and the Secrets of Nature:*

> How are nature's "secrets" to be discovered? The answer is that nature puts a mark on things: the outward appearances of things provides clues or signs pointing to the properties that would otherwise be totally hidden from view. The "signatures" or visual likenesses . . . were not merely coincidences but were divinely ordained. They were woven into the fabric of nature, giving it meaning and intelligibility. Without signatures, nature would be baffling and impenetrable.[3]

The study of Nature's secret messages requires people to observe and use their own outside-the-box thinking to determine what interpretation feels right to them. For example, Steve Jobs, the CEO of Apple, often challenges workers to go beyond their everyday thinking. One day, he was so upset by his employees' lack of creativity that he grabbed a chair and started hammering it against the wall and used so much force that he smashed a hole big enough to see into the next room. He dramatically made his point: there's more beyond the four walls of a room and the "walls" of our minds.

Jobs shook up our reality in order for us to "Think Different," as the Apple slogan goes. This book presents plenty of controversial concepts that are guaranteed to get some people's panties in a bunch. That's good. Why not challenge what we think and know to be "true"? If our original thoughts turn out to be right, that's great . . . but if not, *voilà!* A new understanding is born!

Nature is not one size fits all. She is far too complex to characterize with sweeping generalizations, but if you're willing to test new points of view, you're bound to discover more of her brilliance all around you. You'll be stretching your creativity and sense of wonder at the same time. Think of Nature as a gym or even a playground for your imagination and inner wisdom.

"Our destination is never a place, but rather a new way of looking at things."

— **Henry Miller**

Many of Nature's signs that you'll read about in this book may seem obvious at first, but I've included them because in order to discover the more mysterious signs, you need to start with basic concepts. You must carefully consider the entire plant and its environment, including the flowers, leaves, stems, shapes, colors, roots, scent, and soil. The more closely you observe Nature's works of art, the more likely you are to view something you've never seen. Don't be surprised if you find yourself wondering, *How could I have missed that?*

Do You Have a Signature?

Do you think someone could quickly figure out *your* signature? You may think, *Oh no, I'm much too complex for that! People need to take time to get to know me.* In his book *Blink,* Malcolm Gladwell reports a study in which those who snooped around a person's dorm room for 15 minutes knew more about the individual than their friends. Just like plants, your environment creates a signature that leaves many clues.

Gladwell also writes about a researcher who claims that marriages have signatures. By reading the signs, he can predict (with 95 percent accuracy) if couples will still be married within 15 years by observing one hour of their conversations. Four signs that a marriage is in trouble are contempt, defensiveness, stonewalling, and criticism—with contempt being the worst. This once again shows that there are signs everywhere—in Nature and in us!

The following chapters will explore several simple signs to pique your interest. You can decide for yourself whether Nature offers you insightful messages and love letters or if what you observe is just a bunch of uncanny coincidences. Either way, as you combine your imagination with knowledge, you'll acquire some surprising ways to remember important facts about food. (I *still* remember my kindergarten teacher using ordinary objects to create works of art. Shoe boxes became toy school buses, for example, and Popsicle sticks morphed into toy animals. I remember these more than any other school projects because my teacher activated my imagination.)

Let's begin by looking at how Nature mirrors us.

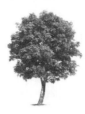

CHAPTER TWO

Nature Is Our Mirror

*"We still do not know one-thousandth of
one percent of what nature has revealed to us."*

— **Albert Einstein**

Take a moment to use your imagination and look at food in ways in which ancient people might have. Long ago, many names of plants and flowers were based on their appearance and characteristics (think eyebright, foxtail, and maidenhair fern, for example). People easily remembered these catchy names and handed them down from generation to generation.

This system is still in use today. Did you know that the Black-Berry PDA got its name because its buttons resemble the berry's seeds? Chances are very good that you'll remember the benefits of most of the following foods that I've highlighted in this chapter—forever and without any effort—if you simply engage a little curiosity and imagination as you read.

"Nut Cases"

Have you ever *really* looked at a walnut? The ancients observed that the meat of the walnut is encased in a hard protective shell, just like the "meat" of the human brain is encased in a hard protective skull. Furthermore, when you break open a walnut shell, the nut inside contains two halves resembling the brain's two hemispheres. When you take the walnut out of the shell, it resembles the brain even more.

The English Walnut	The Brain
Has two equal sides	Has a left and right hemisphere
Encased in a hard protective shell	Encased in a hard protective skull
Covered with furrows	Covered with furrows
Composed of approximately 68 percent of beneficial fat	Composed of approximately 67 percent structural fat and requires beneficial fats from foods to function

Nature's Secret Message

Nature engages our imagination by offering us clues about the benefits of specific foods.

Interestingly, even our language relates this nut to the brain. For example, we say that someone is "driving us nuts," "going nuts," or a "total nutcase."

Ancient people believed that because of the uncanny resemblance, walnuts must be beneficial for the human brain in some way. And this wasn't a nutty concept! Today, walnuts are on many top-ten "superfood" lists because research shows that they contain beneficial omega-3 fats, which support brain function, increase memory, and help manage hyperactivity, depression, and even autism. The body can't manufacture omega-3 fats, so we must get them from food sources such as nuts.

Among almonds, cashews, hazelnuts, macadamia nuts, pistachios, walnuts, and pecans, can you guess which one has the largest amount of brain-enriching omega-3 fats? You've got it—the walnut! And here's another fascinating coincidence: the brain and walnut are both made up of about 68 percent fat. (So if someone calls you a fathead, take it as a compliment!)

Another distinguishing feature of the walnut is its combination of both omega-3 fats and alpha-linolenic acid (ALA), making it one of the few nonfish sources of these essential fats. (Flaxseeds also contain a high amount of ALA.)

And there's more: research further shows that walnuts benefit the heart. According to findings from two large multicenter, randomized studies, these nuts are packed with fatty acids, nutrients, bioactive compounds, phytosterols, and folic acid—all of which may fight against heart disease. Walnuts also contain high levels of L-arginine, an essential amino acid known to help with hypertension, and ellagic acid, which dramatically decreases arteriosclerotic lesions in animals.[1] Walnut oil contains no cholesterol and reduces the formation of new vascular plaque. It's mind-boggling how many nutrients and beneficial fats can fit into one compact shell.

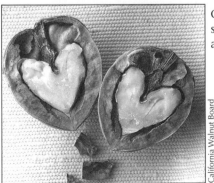

Could the walnut meat's heart shape relate to the fact that it's also a heart-healthy food?

California Walnut Board

Just-for-Fun Quiz!

Test Your Nature IQ

1. What inspired George Washington Carver to develop crop rotation and the many uses for peanuts?

2. How can you absorb eight times more nutrition out of walnuts?

3. Does the human body produce vitamin C?

4. How can you pick the juiciest fruit out of a bunch?

5. Which fruit is mentioned the most times in the Bible?

6. If a plant has a strong smell (and it's not rotting), what might that indicate?

7. Which fruit has its seeds on the outside?

Answers

1. His love of nature watching
2. By soaking them
3. No
4. Juice weighs more than pulp, so choose the heaviest fruit.
5. The fig
6. Plants with strong smells are generally used for medicinal purposes or in ceremonies.
7. The strawberry

Now you might say, "Yeah, but walnuts—and all nuts, for that matter—are really fattening. They have so many calories that I try to avoid them." Let me share a little secret I learned from Ken Blue, the executive chef at the Hippocrates Health Institute in West Palm Beach, Florida: soaking nuts in water breaks down the fats so that your body is less likely to store them as fat—hence making them less fattening.[2]

Here's why: Your body needs enzymes to digest food, and there are enzyme inhibitors on the outside of the nuts to protect them—think of it as Nature's bubble wrap. These inhibitors act like a protective barrier for the walnut, which prevents easy digestion, but soaking nuts in water releases these inhibitors and makes them easier to digest. It also makes them more alkaline and increases their vitality and nutritional value—sometimes up to eight times— because the germination process activates and multiplies the nutrients. Because the body doesn't have to work so hard to digest the nuts, and because they're more nutritious, you get more energy from eating them in this way. (By the way, traditional Chinese doctors say that walnut skin is slightly toxic and should be peeled off so that it doesn't counteract some of the nut's nutritional benefits.)

You may be surprised by how quick and easy it is to soak your walnuts in water—and how noticeably tastier they become! Soaking walnuts—or any nuts or seeds, for that matter—is incredibly simple: just place them in a bowl of water and leave them overnight at room temperature. In the morning, rinse them well and dry thoroughly. Then store the nuts in a container (preferably glass) in the refrigerator. Soak only what you can use in three or four days because they're more likely to attract mold.

You can get them to last longer if you dehydrate them after soaking. (You can do this by placing them in a 118 degree oven for several hours or in an inexpensive commercial dehydrator; see the recommendations in Appendix II). Ken says that removing warm, crunchy nuts from a dehydrator is just like taking fresh cookies out of the oven. They're so tasty . . . you'll go nuts for them!

How Many Walnuts Should You Eat?

In a nutshell, here are some guidelines about walnuts:

- Eating as few as four walnuts four times a week will increase omega-3s in your body and can improve brain function.

- Just a quarter cup of walnuts (about 10–12 halves) provides 90.8 percent of your daily value (DV) for these essential fats.

- According to the U.S. Food and Drug Administration, research suggests that "eating 1.5 ounces [a handful] of walnuts per day, as part of a low saturated fat and low cholesterol diet . . . may reduce the risk of coronary heart disease."[3]

The next secret message from Nature is another no-brainer because (as with walnuts) the food in question looks so much like the body part that it helps.

"See" Food

Take a look at the picture of the sliced carrot on the following page. "I" bet you can tell which body part will benefit from its nutrients. But why are carrots so beneficial for our eyes? The eye-opening truth is that of all the vegetables, carrots contain the highest level of carotene (which converts to vitamin A), and research shows that this helps prevent cataracts and macular degeneration.

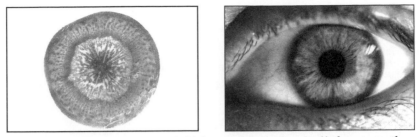

Carrots contain more carotene (which converts to vitamin A) than any other vegetable, and our eyes need vitamin A to help prevent macular degeneration and cataracts.

One carrot is all you need to get 203 percent of the recommended daily allowance (RDA) of vitamin A.[4] *One carrot!* You can eat it raw, cooked, whole, shredded, chopped, sliced, or dipped . . . any way you'd like.

Berry Power

You may have heard that berries are also beneficial for eye health, but they don't look like eyes! A shaman figures it this way: you see in color; therefore, you need colorful foods such as carrots and berries to maintain good vision. It may sound simplistic, but research proves that antioxidants, which protect the body's cells from the damaging effects of oxidation and may help reduce the risk of macular degeneration, are found in the pigments (the color) of food. So the shaman got it *r-eye-t.*

The fundamental rule of the "see food" diet is to choose brightly colored fruits and vegetables, as these are generally known to be the most nutritious. Those that are less vivid have often been picked too soon, so they haven't had enough time to develop vibrant colors—and higher levels of nutrients.

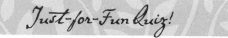

Just-for-Fun Quiz!

Test Your Nature IQ

Question: According to Chinese medicine, which body organ are eye issues associated with?

Answer: The liver. If you experience chronic bloodshot eyes, dry eyes, or blurry vision, consider having your liver checked. (And check out the symptoms of computer vision syndrome that appear a bit further in this chapter.)

For extra credit, guess which organ converts the carotene in carrots to vitamin A (to help the eyes)? You got it—the liver!

It probably won't surprise you to hear that carotene is named after the carrot because of its high levels of carotene, which is what gives it its bright orange color. Generally, the more orange that fruits and vegetables appear, the more carotene they contain. The following chart shows the amounts of vitamin A in some favorite orange-colored foods.[5]

Orange Foods	Amount of Vitamin A	Percent Daily Value of Vitamin A
1 cup raw carrot	21,383 IU	428%
1 cup raw sweet potato	18,866 IU	377%
1 cup raw pumpkin	8,567 IU	171%
1 cup raw cantaloupe	5,987 IU	120%
1 cup raw apricot	2,985 IU	60%

Methods for Naturally Improving Your Vision

A nutritious diet that's chock-full of vitamin A isn't the only way you can maintain healthy eyes. Nature provides additional clues to help you maximize eye health. When you're in a natural setting, your eyes automatically focus on objects both near and far, rather than remaining fixed for long periods on items that are either up close (like a computer screen) or in the distance (such as the road when you're driving in light traffic). By mirroring Nature's way of seeing and varying the distance at which you gaze, you strengthen your vision. Here are some easy, natural eye exercises that may help your vision.

Eye Gym

For more than 30 years, ocular therapist Dawn Rose, founder of the Vision Re-Education Center in San Diego, has helped thousands of people improve their eyesight through specific exercises. According to Rose, your eyes don't have to worsen with age. The eye is a muscle, and just like any other muscle in your body, you lose what you don't use.

One of the simple eye exercises Rose teaches is called "butterfly blinks." Throughout the day, softly flutter your eyelids as if they were light butterfly wings. This will lubricate the surface of your eyes, which will help you see more clearly.[6]

If you suffer from dry eyes, eyestrain, neck and backaches, or even blurred vision, you might have a condition called CVS (computer vision syndrome). This happens when you focus on something that's close to you (such as your computer screen) for very long periods, which weakens eye muscles. Orlin Sorensen, the founder of the Rebuild Your Vision Program, recommends practicing the "10-10-10 rule" while working at a computer: every ten minutes, look ten feet away for ten seconds. Dawn Rose also instructs people to keep looking far away (preferably out to Nature) then near, and vice versa—like doing reps at the gym. (To gently and automatically remind yourself to take a time-out on a regular basis while you're working, you can download a free software program called Time Out by Dejal Systems.)

Eye exercises require about 25 minutes a day, but many people don't spend the time because they don't think of their eyes as "lazy" or "weak." Maybe they'd rather just rely on eyeglasses. Keep in mind that the more you try to "help" Nature with "improvements," the more lazy and dependent you can become. For example, foods that haven't been pampered or protected are healthier because they work harder to protect themselves, thereby increasing their nutrient levels. So consider investing time exercising your eyes. It's the natural way to good vision.

Palming

Another natural way to promote eye health is through the practice of "palming," which stone carvings tell us the ancients used more than 60,000 years ago. Palming brings energy from your hands to your eyes, and Dawn Rose has seen it create positive change in the vision of thousands of people—even those with macular degeneration.

Palming also helps you relax your whole body. After all, Rose claims that 95 percent of the tension in a person's body is held in the eyes.[6] And as you'll see when you try this technique, your palms fit perfectly over your eye sockets—yet another "coincidence" showing us the connection between Nature and your health.

Before you "palm," make sure your hands are clean. Then shake them out to release any tension, and rub the palms of your hands together to create new energy. Gently cup them (without pressing) over your open eyes, with your fingers on your forehead. You should see only darkness. Then with a straight spine and neck, close your eyes. Relax your eyes and notice how your body relaxes, too. Think of happy or appreciative thoughts and memories. Rose suggests palming for one minute every hour, or you can simply try it whenever you feel the need to unwind or center yourself.

Another ancient secret is to have the sun radiate on your *closed* eyes for a few minutes a day to relax your eyes and ease tension. But be sure to do this during the early morning or late afternoon, when the warmth of the sun is therapeutic. During midday, the sun's rays may be too strong.

"C" This One

Another orange-colored food that Nature has coded for us is the orange. Take a closer look at one. What does the texture of the peel resemble to you? When learning to give shots, nurses used to practice on oranges because they look and feel like skin. Given that appearances often relate to a plant's nutritional value, could oranges be good for our skin?

You may have seen advertisements for anti-aging, wrinkle-reducing creams that tout vitamin C as a key ingredient. One popular, pricey skin cream even claims: "Maximum levels of vitamin C provide a firmer, brighter, and overall more youthful appearance." Why is this so? Because research shows that vitamin C supports the development of collagen, which keeps skin firm and reduces the appearance of wrinkles.[7]

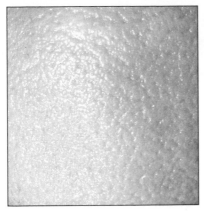

Nature gives us clues to show us that eating vitamin C–packed oranges, which resemble our skin when looked at up close, promotes healthy skin.

The body doesn't produce vitamin C, which is a good reason to include oranges, rich in this nutrient, in your diet. Oranges contain structured water (which penetrates the cells at a faster rate and helps you absorb nutrients more efficiently) as well as beneficial antioxidants. When you improve your cellular health, you see results in your skin because not only is the skin your body's largest organ, but it's also connected to every system in the body.

Nature's Diversity Echoes Our Diversity

You may now want to run right out for some oranges and lotion infused with vitamin C to help improve your skin, but hold it right there. Even in Nature, there's no one-size-fits-all directive because everyone's needs are different. Talk to your doctor or dermatologist to decide what amount of vitamin C *you* need to benefit your skin and overall health. For example, according to the ancient system of Indian medicine called Ayurveda, people fall into one of three categories: Pitta, Vata, and Kapha. Ayurvedic practitioners believe that people who are the Pitta type should avoid citrus, despite its vitamin C content, whereas Vata and Kapha types are fine with it.

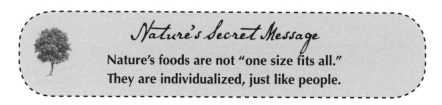

Nature's Secret Message
**Nature's foods are not "one size fits all."
They are individualized, just like people.**

The theory that some foods are beneficial for some people and not for others may explain why some people can lose weight on a particular diet, while others will either stay the same weight or even gain pounds on the same plan. So how do you tell which foods are good for you and will enhance your own physical health? It's kind of like when you choose friends. You find who is best for you by hanging out and noting your experiences. You quickly realize that you get along with some people better than others.

You can do the same thing to see which food agrees with you the most by keeping a food journal and writing about how you feel a few hours after your meal. If you feel tired, irritable, sad, or generally unwell, you might have eaten something that doesn't agree with you. It takes some investigative work and yes, some time, but the results are worth it. Soon you may come to realize that a certain food can change your energy levels or even your personality. For example, a high-school girl I counseled told me that she was unhappy and believed that depression was just her lot in life. I asked her to keep a food journal and when I looked at what she ate, I calculated that she was consuming more than 40 teaspoons of sugar per day. It was *a lot* of sugar, not her lot in life, that was making her depressed!

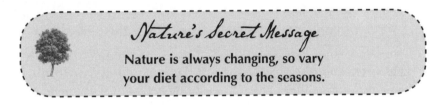

Nature's Secret Message
**Nature is always changing, so vary
your diet according to the seasons.**

So even though many of the tips you'll read here are backed up by scientific studies, it's still wise to check which ones are good for you and your unique body. Keep in mind, too, that just as Nature changes and varies foods according to the seasons, you can benefit by doing the same. What's great for you in winter may not be especially good for you in summer. You can tune in to your body and let it decide whether a particular food is beneficial for you at a certain time.

Here's a simple way to use the wisdom of your own body to check whether a particular food or supplement is good for you. Hold the item in question to your chest. Close your eyes, tune in to your inner wisdom, and ask, "Is this beneficial for me?" Note which way your body seems to sway or lean. Test several foods in this way, including ones that you know aren't good for you. Write down your answers. Generally, if your body moves forward, it means that the food is a good one for you; if you find yourself leaning backward, it's a signal that you should avoid this item.

If your body doesn't seem to be moving in a distinct way, test the food again, asking whether eating a large amount of it would be good for you. If you ask, "Will drinking the entire bottle of this be good for me?" this extreme example could cause your body to respond by gravitating forward or backward. You might also ask how much you should eat.

This method can take a bit of practice, so keep experimenting with it to see if it works for you. It's just one of many tools to access your intuition and body wisdom. (Another popular method is called applied kinesiology used by many chiropractors, which evaluates structural, chemical, and mental aspects of health using manual muscle testing [biofeedback from the body] with other standard methods of diagnosis.)

The Avocado—Pregnant with Possibility

Let's consider the avocado next. What message do you think it might hold? Remember to focus on its appearance. Take a pregnant pause to think about this one. If you look closely at the avocado's unusual shape, you'll see that it resembles the torso of a pregnant woman. And if you cut one open, you'll see that it contains an unusually large seed. A pregnant woman also has a large "seed" inside. Could the avocado, then, contain anything that's specifically beneficial for pregnant women?

An Avocado	A Pregnant Woman
Contains a large seed inside	Carries her baby in the womb
Has a distinctive shape, larger and rounder toward the bottom	Develops a large, rounded belly
Is loaded with healthy fat, which supports cell growth	Accumulates fat to support her baby and herself throughout pregnancy and after birth
Contains more of the antioxidant lutein than any other fruit[8]	Produces increased amounts of lutein that's transferred into breast milk and umbilical-cord plasma.[9] (Researchers aren't sure why yet, but lutein is believed to benefit both mother and child.)
Contains about 74 percent water; these thirsty trees require more water than most others	Requires more water intake than usual

Since the avocado is so smooth, it's one of the first foods babies can eat. It also contains high levels of potassium, which is beneficial for relieving stress and anxiety, as well as the cramps some women experience with their menstrual cycle.

The Birth of a New Perspective

According to the California Avocado Commission, a medium-sized avocado has 22.5 grams of fat. Healthy fats are critical for pregnant women and their unborn babies because not eating enough of this fat can raise the risk of premature birth and even postnatal depression. Fat also plays an important role in fertility. Women with low body fat may miss menstrual periods and struggle with fertility issues.

Do you avoid avocados because you think they're fattening? The avocado, highly regarded for thousands of years, fell out of popularity during the low-fat diet craze, but the ancients had it right. Approximately 80 percent of the 400 calories in an eight-ounce avocado come from the oil, which is the *healthy*, monounsaturated kind of fat.

Living in Southern California, I've attended many raw food "un-cooking" classes that call for avocados in dishes. I've noticed that the people who attend these classes aren't overweight—in fact, some are too thin! It's unfortunate that many people ignore this healthy, tasty fruit for fear of its calories, but they don't think twice about eating junk food or man-made foods loaded with chemicals because they are considered to be "low calorie" or "reduced fat." All calories are not alike. If we reorient our food attention to focus on Nature's food versus synthetics, we can be healthier, leaner, and happier.

Choosing the Best Avocado

The avocado has a buttoned-up secret. If you remove the button from the top of the fruit and the color underneath is green, it's ripe and ready to eat. But if you spot any brown or yellow, it's not ready yet.

Avocado farmer Bradley Miles of Carpinteria, California, says that if there's no button, insects have an easy entrance into the fruit. Also, an avocado with no button is a sign that it may not be as good as the others, since those could be the ones that fell to the ground instead of being cut from the tree.[10]

Now let's look at the pomegranate, which gives us a clue *before* it falls to the ground.

Don't Take the Pomegranate for Granted

Throughout time, the succulent pomegranate has symbolized abundance, fruitfulness, life, and female energy. Because of its many seeds, it has long been a symbol of fertility. Leonardo da Vinci, Paul Cézanne, Salvador Dalí, and Sandro Botticelli all included the pomegranate in their paintings.

When buying this fruit, how do you know which one is ripe? Farmer Gene Etheridge of Etheridge Farms located in Dinuba, California, has been observing the growth and ripening of pomegranates for more than 18 years. He noticed that if a pomegranate is left alone, the fruit will eventually split open and all the seeds will drop to the ground. Before it "gives birth," however, it develops stretch marks, just like a pregnant woman does. Etheridge says that's a message to pick it *now,* before it splits open. So look for a pomegranate with stretch marks—it will be a ripe one.[11]

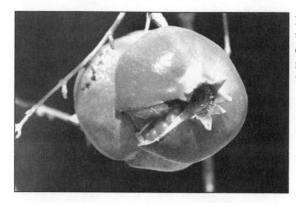

Nature mirrors us. Pomegranates develop "stretch marks" before "birthing" seeds.

One thing is for sure: We don't need to stretch our imagination to know that the pomegranate is one nutritious fruit. The ancients believed rich red foods helped the blood and heart, and in this case, it's true. Numerous studies have proven that the pomegranate is a heart-healthy food that fights inflammation, improves blood flow, decreases LDL (the "bad" cholesterol), and reduces the growth of arterial plaque.[12]

As long as we've been discussing pregnancy, let's look at a food that's more than 60 million years old and has been associated with sex, fertility, procreation, maternal nourishment, and can also grow in pairs. Can you guess what food it is?

Figs—Meant for Your Imagination

Like the pomegranate, the fig is highly alkaline, packed with nutrients and numerous seeds. Many different cultures have associated these seeds with life and fertility. In fact, in ancient Egypt, anyone pruning the fig tree was thought to be risking sterility. The fig is also the most mentioned fruit in the Bible.

What makes the fig tree unusual is that unlike most trees that have leaves, grow flowers, and then bear fruit, the fig tree first has figs, then leaves, but never flowers, as they are invisible within the fig.[13]

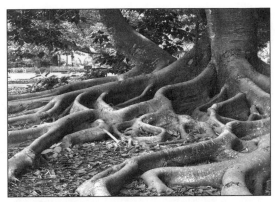

Exotic roots of a bay fig tree. With a lineage of 60 million years, flexibility, adaptability, and resilience are the fig's secrets to survival.

According to fig-grower Lloyd Kreitzer, known as "the Fig Man," figs break all of Nature's rules and even play dead while other plants are blooming. Kreitzer believes figs do things differently because they're from ancient times. You may not have thought twice about figs, but imagine being able to trace your family "tree" back over 60 million years like you can with this unique tree.

Figs have *fig*ured out that having flexibility, adaptability, patience, and resilience are what's helped them to survive. One farmer reported how a strong wind blew a cage onto a fig tree and knocked it to the ground, where it lay entirely on its side, apparently ruined. When he finally went to discard the tree a few weeks later, he was amazed to find that it not only survived, but later that season it bore fruit as if nothing had happened and continued to thrive. There's much we can learn from Nature!

Kreitzer first became interested in this fruit when his body broke out in painful boils from inoculations he'd received upon entering the Peace Corps. He tried everything to heal them and eventually found that placing the seedy side of a fig (especially if it had been heated) onto the boil and wrapping the area in an Ace bandage gave him the greatest relief.[13]

Kreitzer isn't the first person to have picked up on this connection between figs and boils. Paul Pitchford, in his book *Healing with Whole Foods,* states that figs can be applied to skin discharges and boils.[14] Maybe they help heal these conditions because they contain chemicals called psoralens that have been used for thousands of years to treat skin pigmentation diseases. Figs have a high mineral content, which can benefit the skin.

You can make a tasty hors d'oeuvre with figs by serving them with melted goat cheese or tossing them into a fresh salad. And while you're thinking about salad, you might want to consider the special benefits of one of those delicious greens: Swiss chard.

The Secrets of Swiss Chard

Take a close look at a piece of Swiss chard, as its appearance provides several clues to its value for your body. Notice that all those rich red veins resemble the circulatory system. Also consider that the color green is associated with the heart chakra. Numerous studies have proven that eating greens benefits the heart. Research reveals that chard is loaded with beneficial phenolic antioxidants and kaempferol, which help to prevent arteriosclerosis and inhibit plaque formation. Green leafy plants, including Swiss chard, are a great source of chlorophyll, a known blood builder.

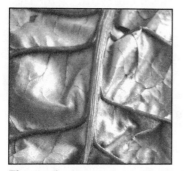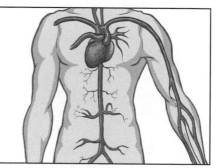

The similar appearance of Swiss chard "veins" [left] and our circulatory system could be Nature's way of telling us that chard benefits our body.

Juicing: The Fountain of Youth?

A great way to add Swiss chard and greens to your diet is to put them through a juicer with other vegetables to make what I call a "miracle" drink. Simply juice lots of greens, add an apple for sweetness, and maybe toss in a little lemon and ginger for zing. Yum!

Juicing veggies may not sound tasty, but I've met junk-food lovers who became hooked on this miracle drink. I've also personally witnessed people dramatically change in appearance, mood, and energy level just by drinking *fresh* juices. This occurred when I worked on a TV pilot in which participants were allowed to consume only fresh vegetable juices for two weeks. I met everyone the day they started and didn't see them again until the two-week cleanse ended. I was amazed at their dramatic transformation in such a short period of time! When I first saw one of the participants, I actually wondered if it was the same person.

Consuming the vital life force in green plants—especially *dark* green plants—leads to radiant skin and a calm demeanor. People who drink green juice consistently rave about its ability to detoxify, alkalize, and invigorate the body, as well as cleanse the blood and increase circulation. It's no wonder their skin glows and their bodies are energized!

Reading the Messages from Our Bodies

"What is always speaking silently is the body."

— Norman O. Brown

Just as we can learn to look at a plant and discern some of its properties from its appearance, we can also learn to "read" our bodies for deeper messages. Few are more skilled at this than Johnny Seitz, a life coach, professional ballet dancer and choreographer,

31

internationally recognized mime, and adult with autism. He has also taught at Harvard and New York University and is the author of the book *Bio-Typing Beyond Body Language.* Because of Seitz's exceptional sensitivity and heightened awareness, he's able to help people with seemingly unsolvable emotional and physical issues with regard to strokes, autism, and depression. He can determine the deeply rooted, subconscious truths behind people's actions by observing their body's clues—in other words, he's able to see what's *hidden in plain sight.*

Seitz explains that there's a secret language behind human movements. Everyone has learned to read basic body language to some extent. For example, we can easily interpret a loved one's relaxed muscles and open arms as a sign that affection is welcome, versus a tense posture and crossed arms and legs that communicate, "Keep your distance!" But Seitz contends that this is just the tip of the iceberg.

He states that the same "muscle methodology" that people use to hold their bodies upright and to move in certain ways is exactly the same methodology they use to deal with situations in other areas of their lives—that is, how someone does one thing is generally how he or she does everything. "The way you approach and solve problems and the way you take in information is predicated on how you feel and think—which is reflected in the body," he explains.[15] Yoga teaches that "a flexible spine is a flexible mind." The inverse can also be true: "A rigid spine is a rigid mind."

Your body does more talking than even your own words. Think of how depressed people may have bent-over posture and restricted breathing. Seitz concludes: "Show me how your body reacts to stress, and I'll show you how you handle mental and/or emotional stress in your life. Same goes for finding balance."[15] How you do one thing is how you do everything.

Interpreting Our Body's Movements

One way in which Seitz gathers clues about people is by watching how they walk. He has identified three walking patterns, each reflecting a different personality style. Each type has advantages and disadvantages—there's no best technique. To determine which type you are, imagine a line on the floor and then walk with your heels touching the line. Next walk with your feet about two inches apart from the line. Finally, walk with your feet shoulder-width apart. The way that feels natural will be your type; the other two will feel awkward. It's easy to tell which one you are when you look down while walking on a treadmill.

Here are Seitz's brief descriptions of what these three types mean:

— If you walk with your heels on the line, feet turned outward, you have the ability to multitask and tend to jump into life's challenges and experiences. You're always ready for action. You focus on the end result, not on the steps to get there, and you address challenges as they appear. You're goal-orientated, a visionary, and have the ability to see others' viewpoints.

— If you walk with your feet parallel about two inches apart from the line, like walking on railroad tracks, you are independent and tend to go places in a step-by-step, logical manner. You don't like to be rushed. You're an efficient planner and organizer, an analytical thinker who observes and studies a situation before making a decision.

— If you walk with your feet shoulder-width apart, you are more of the "I know what I want" type. You have strong opinions, and you tend to be immovable, yet you can make a huge shift when you're ready. You know who you are, and you prefer not to take risks, and live mainly in the present.[15]

As Seitz's body typing illustrates, you can learn infinitely more about yourself—as well as about anything in Nature—through close observation. Watching the way someone walks yields just one of many possible clues. After studying with Seitz, I see how the body is screaming out important messages, but many of us just don't notice. Perhaps if we tune in more often, we'll be more likely to pick out Nature's secret messages, too.

Next let's look at the clues that Nature could be giving us with regard to the heart and how to live in a more heart-centered manner.

"The heart has reasons which Reason does not know."

— **Blaise Pascal**

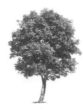

CHAPTER THREE

The Heart of the Matter

*"Deep in the human unconsciousness is a pervasive
need for a logical universe that makes sense. But the
real universe is always one step beyond logic."*

— **Frank Herbert**

I recently came across a picture of a microscopic view of my blood cells, taken during a blood-cell test I had done years ago. As I stared at the photo, I was struck by how much the cells looked like grapes. *Is there a connection?* I wondered.

As it turns out, there is. Science tells us that two chemicals in grapes, resveratrol and polyphenol, help reduce the risk factors for coronary heart disease. In addition, resveratrol is touted as a particularly powerful anti-aging agent. Let's look further and see if there are more clues.

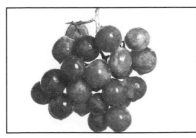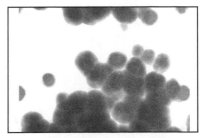

Grapes [left] resemble blood cells [microscopic view, at right] and contain resveratrol and polyphenols, which are known to help the heart and blood.

Signs of the Vines

Indigenous people knew that the shape of a plant, fruit, or food might contain an important clue as to its benefit for humans. For example, they noticed how a vine's stems spread out, a characteristic not shared by other plants, and asked themselves, *What spreads out that way in the body?*

They decided that the vines resembled veins that circulate blood throughout the body. So long before we ever knew about the resveratrol, polyphenols, and antioxidants in grapes—all of which foster healthy blood—ancient civilizations intuited that grapes were food for the blood.

Even a cluster of grapes on a stem resembles the shape of a human heart . . . don't you think? With a little help from your imagination, it certainly does!

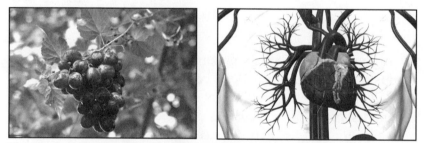

The similarity between a cluster of grapes [left] and the heart [right] could be another clue for us compliments of Mother Nature.

We all know that human hearts aren't truly "heart shaped," and no one's quite certain where the symbolic heart shape originated, but it's speculated that it represents the lines of a woman's curved breasts coming around and down to a point at the vulva. Whatever the ancients might have known about the connection between the actual and symbolic shape and color of the heart, it's fascinating to see how plants that mimic the symbolic heart shape are often beneficial for the actual heart.

Because ancient civilizations took time to observe a plant's external characteristics in order to look for clues to the medicinal potential within, they took note of the large heart-shaped leaves of the Sangre de Drago ("blood of the dragon") and noticed the astonishing similarity between human blood and the dark red sap oozing out of the tree's bark. They took this as a sign of its ability to heal wounds and other blood-related issues.

Unbeknownst to each other, people in Brazil, the Dominican Republic, Mexico, and Peru all used this same remedy. How could they have come to the same understanding without communicating with each other? Well, they were all able to discern that the tree's heart-shaped leaves and red sap resembled a heart and blood.

This may sound simplistic, but science now confirms the validity of this indigenous wisdom. Studies prove that the Sangre de Drago sap stimulates fibroblasts and cellular repair, which helps heal wounds and stops bleeding.[1] It contains taspine, which is documented as having anti-inflammatory and antiviral properties.[2] Another chemical in this plant, dimethylcedrusine, not only helps heal wounds—up to four times faster, according to a study done on rats—but it also regenerates skin by producing new collagen. In addition, the sap accelerates healing by acting like a second skin, drying quickly and forming a protective barrier for the wound.[1] Used topically, it supports the regeneration of healthy tissue with minimal scarring.

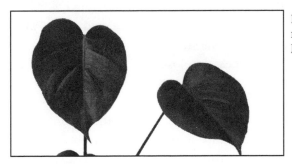

Have you ever noticed heart-shaped leaves in Nature?

Other trees may have similar heart-shaped leaves and red sap, but in this case we know that the Sangre de Drago's benefits were discovered by the insightful observations of people who were tuned in to Nature—people who were astoundingly correct!

What happens when the flow of blood from your heart to your lungs is obstructed? You turn blue. The Aztecs and Chinese, independently, used this observation when contemplating the blue heart-shaped flower of the *Commelina pallida* plant. They interpreted these characteristics to mean that the flowers could be used to constrict or stop the flow of blood.[3]

Does this sound like a stretch? In the late 19th century, the National Medical Institute of Mexico investigated the plant, tested it on the jugular vein of pigeons, and found that it could indeed contract the vein until circulation was cut off completely. Other tests confirmed that the plant coagulates blood and has vasoconstrictor effects, just as ancient people concluded centuries before.[4]

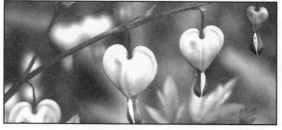

Take a guess . . . which emotional remedy is this plant used for?

Nature's Bleeding Hearts

The delicate red bleeding-heart flower is aptly named, with its "teardrop" clinging to the bottom of a heart-shaped bud. Plant essences and homeopathic remedies made from these poppy plants (*Dicentra spectabilis;* Papaveraceae) are used to cleanse the heart as well as address emotional pain and sadness—the very emotions the flower evokes!

Opinions differ about whether this flower can actually help with emotional issues. A German scientific journal noted that no studies back up the claims that this flower helps with heart issues. However, research is costly, and if it's unlikely to lead to patentable, profitable results, it's not practical to invest the money it takes to explore the plant's potential healing abilities. After all, you can't patent the bleeding-heart plant, and no patent equals no profit.

It's important to keep in mind the limitations of research when considering those who claim that the plant wisdom of indigenous people hasn't been validated by laboratory findings. However, in this case, we do have some evidence. In Chinese medicine, certain chemical compounds from the bleeding-heart plant are used to stimulate the blood with its cardiovascular actions. Bleeding heart is also a popular homeopathic and flower-essence remedy taken for help in loving others unconditionally and with an open heart.

Working with Nature's Energy via Energetic Essences

Flower essences are liquid, energetic remedies derived from live flowers. David Dalton, the founder and director of Delta Gardens, a company that produces a wide array of flower essences, explains that they can be used to heal physical, emotional, and mental imbalances. He claims that "because of their energetic and living quality, they work directly and deeply in the emotional system, assisting in the release of early wounding and trauma. These early imprints, suppressed within the emotional system, are considered one of the main causes of many types of disease and imbalance."[5]

Flower essences can be taken orally, massaged onto the hands and feet, added to drinking water, or sprayed into the air from a misting bottle. Adults, children, and pets can all benefit from them; yet everyone responds to this treatment differently. According to Dalton, "For some, the results are immediate and quite dramatic; for others, the shift is subtle and gradual. Over a period of time, however, flower essences can produce deep and profound changes in the psyche."[5] Therefore, he stresses, if you take them, you should seek the guidance of a flower-essence expert.

Remember that the heart-shaped walnuts, which we discussed earlier, have been scientifically proven to be heart healthy. Another heart-shaped plant is motherwort (*Leonurus cardiaca*), which is used as a heart tonic and also helps relieve symptoms of menopause.

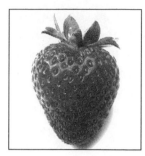

A sensual, heart-shaped strawberry has romantic appeal and contains heart-healthy phenols.

Sensual, red, heart-shaped strawberries, a member of the rose family, are known throughout the ages for their romantic appeal. Strawberries not only look like the heart, but they're also famous for their phenol content, an anti-inflammatory that makes them heart protective.

Nature's Secret Message

Some foods and plants that benefit the heart may actually resemble this organ (or the circulatory system), either visually or metaphorically.

The Heart as a Metaphor

"The heart has a way of knowing what the mind can never know."

— **Mahatma Gandhi**

Is Nature giving us heartfelt messages? There's a story about God hiding the secrets of life so they'd be safe. Where's the last place someone would look? The Almighty searched all over the world, from the highest mountain to the deepest waters, looking for the best spot. Finally, he came up with the perfect place: deep inside our hearts.

The human heart stores tremendous amounts of love and wisdom. Even our language expresses "heartfelt" gestures, meaning something of cherished value. But could the heart *shape* in Nature, known widely throughout the world and across great spans of time, hold wisdom for us also?

When you point to yourself, referring to who you are, you don't point to your head . . . you point to your heart. When people say, "I know it by heart," they mean that it's second nature to them. The heart has been referred to as a "house with many mansions," meaning that the heart houses depths of wisdom and compassion.

According to psychotherapist Len Worley, Ph.D., the heart is the seat of courage and wisdom. Remarkable changes occur in your body when you gently breathe, imagining that your breath is flowing in and out of your heart. Immune function increases, blood pressure is lowered, and digestion improves. Placing your attention on this pleasant form of breathing reduces stress and enhances your problem-solving ability.

Worley adds that focusing on virtues like gratitude, kindness, or humility (where deeper wisdom lies) while practicing heart-focused breathing can literally create a psychoactive response in your brain's neurochemistry, acting like a natural Prozac. Sending courage, love, appreciation, or any other positive emotion to your heart can shift you out of mundane thinking and into the discovery of the hidden secrets of life that are just waiting to be uncovered. What's more, this practice helps you connect with others.[6]

Architect and meditation teacher Michael Meissner suggests that you simply close your eyes, breathe in surrender and acceptance into your heart, and breathe out forgiveness and gratitude.[7] These are the qualities of the four chambers of the heart. Watch and listen as you sit in the great company of your own loving heart, which knows things that the mind can't even begin to understand. When you're near to your heart, you're never far from home.

🍃 🍃 🍃   🍃 🍃 🍃

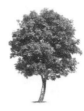

CHAPTER FOUR

Nature—Coming to Your Senses

"Nature does nothing uselessly."

— **Aristotle**

Instead of taking my friend's dog for a walk, I take him for a "stand"—since I stand around while he stops to sniff every bush. His keen sense of smell allows him to read the messages of other animals: he's checking his "pee-mail."

Like my friend's dog, most animals rely on this sense to track down prey, attract mates, and find out who else has been in the area. Sharks are able to detect blood more than a mile away, and deer rub their antlers against tree trunks and branches to leave a scent for potential mates. And I guess size doesn't matter with mountain gorillas—they use their sense of smell to judge the sexual status of other gorillas.

Nature's Secret Message
A strong-smelling plant may mean that it can be used for medicinal or ritual purposes.

Stinkers

Nature often speaks to us through our senses to grab our attention. The Zuni Indians believed that if a plant was strong smelling or noxious, it meant that it was powerful, so they used it both medicinally and in rituals for healing. Generally, studies show that pungent spices also have therapeutic properties. Most of the spices we have in our kitchen have been used medicinally, and their biological activity has been well documented.[1]

Too many studies exist proving the health benefits of odorous garlic to mention here. A grandmother from India was convinced that her swollen, tender gums were healed by keeping a piece of garlic in her mouth between her cheek and gum. And when her granddaughter scraped her gums with a toothbrush and developed a sore, she put garlic on it, which stung momentarily, but soon the pain and sore were gone. Research even shows that the sulfides in garlic may help prevent cancer.

Raw organic garlic, oil of oregano, and tea-tree oil all smell strong, and they are all used to treat a wide array of fungal infections. Sage also has a powerful fragrance that has long been used for ceremonial practices by several cultures. Native Americans use the smoke from burning sage to energetically purify people and objects, and feng shui (the Chinese art of creating harmony and prosperity in a home or building) relies on burning sage to clear negative energy in spaces as well.

My friend even used a natural, nontoxic, foul-smelling potion to get rid of her daughter's head lice. I pictured the lice jumping off her head, holding their noses! This smelly remedy (and others) is guaranteed by the company Topanga Alchemy to remove lice and repel mosquitoes . . . another example of how Nature's "stinkers" are clues from Mother Nature to bring us to our senses!

Durian, called the caviar of fruit, tastes like a rich, creamy custard. However, it gives off such an unpleasant stench that once while I was eating it at a Whole Foods Market, another customer exclaimed, "There's a gas leak!" Stinky as it is, it's a decadent, yummy fruit that has zero saturated fat and plenty of B and C vitamins. A clue from Nature: when it smells bad, it can be *so* good! There's an exception, though: when the scent of a food *changes*, it's letting you know that it's aging and going bad.

Not Smelling Like a Rose

Have you ever wondered if store-bought flowers are losing their fragrance? Flower breeders now have to focus on achieving a longer vase life, as the flowers are usually transported across great distances. In an article published by professors from the University of Michigan and Purdue University, they noted that: "Unfortunately, floral scent has been a casualty of plant-breeding programs for the cut-flower market and ornamental plants in general. . . . Breeders in this multi-billion dollar industry have concentrated on producing plants with improved vase life, shipping characteristics and visual aesthetic values (i.e. color and shape)."[2] After all, what good are great-smelling flowers if they wilt before you buy them? What was once bred for smell is now bred for sell.

The Sounds of Nature

Go in Nature.
Sit still.
Close your eyes.
Listen.

When you tune in to the sounds of Nature, you may be surprised by how quiet and peaceful she can be. Occasionally, you'll hear the song of a bird or the gentle sighing of tree branches overhead. Ever notice how the sound of the leaves trembling in the wind is so different from the sound of the wind whistling through pine trees? As you become more aware of Nature's sounds, you turn down the volume of your "monkey mind," which scampers about from thought to thought.

If you're near a creek, listen to the soothing sound of water as it bubbles over rocks. What other sounds draw you closer to Nature? Does the deep croaking of a frog touch your heart? Do the songs of various birds compete for your attention? Even the buzzing bee takes on a different character when you're relaxed in Nature.

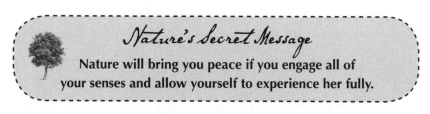

Nature's Secret Message
Nature will bring you peace if you engage all of your senses and allow yourself to experience her fully.

When you're ready to leave a natural setting, allow yourself to hear the dried leaves crunch underfoot with each step you take, a sound you may have missed before. This seemingly simple (and free) exercise of using your senses can be powerful and therapeutic.

Natural sounds are healing in and out of Nature. David Jubb, Ph.D., an author, researcher, and innovator in the field of neurology, claims that listening to the chirping of crickets affects our DNA, and falling asleep to the sound of rain will help drain our lymphatic system (which is responsible for removing excess fluid, waste, and toxins from our body). On the other hand, man-made sounds in the home, such as a television or radio and the humming of the refrigerator, furnace, air conditioner, and other appliances, can have adverse effects on us. Studies show that children actually learn less when exposed to constant, extraneous noises.[3]

Further research proves that loud equipment deeply affects not only our hearing, but also the morale of workers in factories. In addition, scientists are discovering that thanks to a tenfold increase in noisy engines and the waters being more populated by ships than ever before, the auditory onslaught is actually causing fish to secrete 80 to 120 percent more cortisol—the stress hormone.[4] They, like us, are agitated and stressed out by man-made sounds.

In some cases, however, creatures of the sea are using our noise pollution to their advantage. My father manufactures a sound suppressor for machinery used in factories and ships, and his company added their noise dampeners to fishing boats when it was discovered that whales were using the ship's hydraulic noise as a dinner bell! Get this: the ships send out miles of fishing lines with hooks. Once the fish take the bait, the fishermen turn on a noisy hydraulic machine in order to reel in the heavy lines. This noise instantly attracts whales that eat all the fish on the line and know to leave the heads so they won't become caught in the hooks. Once noise suppressors were installed, the sound that attracted the whales was eliminated and the fish were successfully reeled in.

We're not necessarily aware of the myriad noises that affect us because sound is a vibration that our bodies can also pick up subconsciously. Some people even believe that our thoughts create subtle sound vibrations that go out into the universe. What we know for sure, though, is that Nature offers us something for our senses that is so simple, yet so powerfully therapeutic: *peace*. Even when many of Nature's sounds occur together—such as crickets, birds, and frogs in a rural pond setting, or the many animals of the rain forest announcing the sunrise—they create a soothing symphony.

How to Tune Into Nature's Sounds

Getting out into Nature is a perfect way to tune in to her tranquil sounds. However, you can also experience them indoors. Dr. Jubb recommends using a water fountain to bring the sounds of the natural world into your home.[3] It provides soothing white noise, which contains all frequencies and can mask out unwanted sounds, reducing the startle reflex that's a natural response to sudden noises. A wall or garden fountain has the added benefit of producing negative ions that refresh and contribute to your sense of well-being. By the way, you can adjust the sound by increasing or decreasing the amount of water that's flowing, and adding or moving any objects inside the fountain.

Now H*ear* This

"God speaks to us every day, only we don't know how to listen."

— **Mahatma Gandhi**

Notice the similarities between the shape of the ears and kidneys and in how they function. You hear with your ears, but they also filter out noise and dirt. The liquid in the inner-ear canals keeps you balanced. Likewise, the kidneys filter out waste materials and balance the liquid in the body.

Just as the cochlea of the inner ear is spiral shaped, so are the seeds derived from the plant *Cocculus carolinus,* explains Stephen Stiteler, O.M.D., who practices homeopathy and Oriental medicine in Los Angeles. He adds that this plant is the most effective homeopathic remedy for vertigo and dizziness.[5]

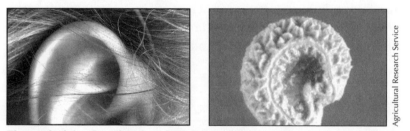

The seed of the *Cocculus* plant [right] resembles the ear and helps treat vertigo.

Dying for Great Taste

Japanese diners could literally get a killer meal if they order the puffer fish known as "fugu." If the chef prepares this delicacy correctly, using only a minute amount of the neurotoxin tetrodotoxin that's naturally found in the fish, diners get a meal that teases their tastes buds and seduces their mouths with tingling and numbing sensations.

However, if prepared incorrectly, this risky fish could cost them their lives. The tetrodotoxin in this fish is 1,200 times deadlier than cyanide. "Tora-fugu" is known to be the most poisonous and most delicious of all puffer fish.

By the way, if a predator tries to catch the puffer fish, it blows itself up to many times its natural size, which startles the predator, allowing the fish to escape. Nature is pretty smart. As to the diners ordering this fish . . . that's yet to be determined.

The puffer fish may not seem appetizing to you, but some of the following foods might. In her infinite wisdom, Mother Nature created six different taste sensations that contain specific health benefits:

1. **Bitter:** Dandelion greens, Swiss chard, radishes, arugula, dulse, endive, turmeric, kale, and ume plum are all bitter. They help your body digest, detoxify, and alkalize (soothing heartburn). These bitter foods can also reduce inflammation and keep your liver healthy.

2. **Pungent:** Gingerroot, garlic, hot peppers, balsamic vinegar, red onions, and spicy foods heat your body, drain sinuses, promote and stimulate circulation, improve absorption of food, and energize you.

3. **Astringent:** Pomegranates, cucumbers, Brussels sprouts, cranberry juice, yellow lentils, cruciferous vegetables (such as cauliflower and cabbage), kidney beans, mung beans, lima beans, and pinto beans all absorb water. You should avoid them if you experience cardiac pain or constipation, but you may find them useful to alleviate diarrhea or excessive bleeding.

4. **Sweet:** Fruits, rice, and honey (eaten in moderation) not only taste good but can also be calming, and can cleanse tissues. (Avoid white processed sugar, which can create havoc in the body.)

5. **Sour:** Lemon, tamarind, grapefruit, sauerkraut, pickles, and yogurt help your liver and nervous system stay healthy.

6. **Salty:** *Un*processed salt (like sea salt), cheeses, and hydrated seaweed can help your kidneys and endocrine system—not to mention add flavor to food.

Because we tend to favor sweet, salty, and sour flavors, consider adding more bitter, astringent, and pungent foods to your diet. This will create a healthy balance and can promote weight loss when necessary.

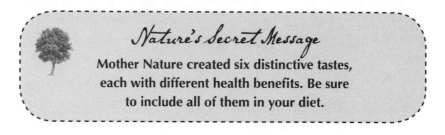

Nature's Secret Message

Mother Nature created six distinctive tastes, each with different health benefits. Be sure to include all of them in your diet.

Now let's see the ways in which Nature's colors can influence your life.

Nature: In Living Color

Color choice can mean life, death, or sex in Nature—it's that important. Many animals and insects are able to change their colors to camouflage themselves and avoid a predator's attack. A butterfly can close its wings to look like a dead, drab leaf to fool a hungry bird looking for a meal, and it can open up and reveal its brilliant colors to strut its stuff.

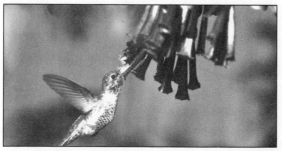

Vibrant colors attract humming-birds. Their beaks match the trumpet shape of the flowers; they're made for each other!

Resembling a hopping singles' bar, Nature graces her creatures with alluring "makeup" to help them attract mates or pollinators. Since color is vital in Nature, let's see how it can help you.

Nature's Vibrant Billboards

Let Mother Nature's paintbrush color your life. She delights in artistically creating food in a variety of colors. She does nothing without good reason, which led me to think, *Could various colors have secret messages?* I suddenly had a hunch while counseling a person who was stuck in a dull rut. "Do you eat only bland-looking food?" I asked. Sure enough, when we reviewed his diet, it consisted of mainly the same colorless foods.

Could your life change by eating more colorful foods? In the documentary *Simply Raw: Reversing Diabetes in 30 Days,* diabetics were able to go off all of their medications in one month by changing their diets to include rich, colorful, live foods. Scientists know that various food colors contain different nutrients. For example, reds generally contain more lycopene, oranges more carotene, blues more anthocyanins, and so on. And the brighter- and darker-colored fruits and vegetables are usually far richer in antioxidants.

Nature's Secret Message

All of the colors in the spectrum are balanced, and Nature offers this same balance in our foods. To maintain optimal health, we must include a colorful variety in our diet.

Color Me "Buddha-ful"—the Energy of Color

Each chakra (energy centers in the body) is associated with a color and a corresponding sound, and every color is a different wavelength of light, which gives it a unique energy. Therefore, since each color has a different tone, eating a variety of colorful foods is like a symphony playing in your body. If you want to be in harmony, give your body a healthy balance of colorful foods. On the other hand, eating the same things every day is like playing "Chopsticks" over and over and won't do much for your body.

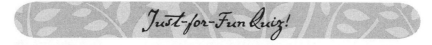

Just-for-Fun Quiz!

Test Your Nature IQ

Try answering these colorful questions:

1. What's the best color plate to use if you're on a diet?

2. What color indicates that a plant or food may contain sunscreening benefits?

3. According to Chinese medicine, what do yellow foods help in the body?

4. Name the color that Leonardo da Vinci is referring to in this quote: "The power of meditation can be ten times greater under _____ light falling through a stained-glass window of a quiet church."

Answers

1. Blue
2. Red
3. The liver and digestion
4. Violet

Like food, color isn't a one-size-fits-all affair. As in life, there are exceptions to the rules, but here are *general* clues of food colors that can help you:

Red. Primitive cultures believed that red food helped the blood, since it mirrors its appearance. We know that beets have a plentiful supply of iron, which nourishes the blood, along with fiber, which helps reduce serum cholesterol. Betacyanin, the red pigment of beets, can increase the blood's oxygen-carrying ability by being absorbed into the blood's corpuscles. The powerful antioxidant lycopene, found in red foods like tomatoes (which even have four chambers like the heart), reduces cholesterol. Anthocyanins, pigments found in many red, blue, and purple fruits, also protect against heart disease.

In a study published in 2005 in *New Scientist* magazine, Cornell University doctoral student YiFan Chu asserts that Red Delicious apple extracts can help prevent oxidation of "bad" cholesterol, which he claims isn't bad until it oxidizes. If Chu's lab experiments are also true for humans eating apples, then eating four could reduce cholesterol levels in the blood by the same amount as one dose of statin drugs.[6] Experiments by pharmacologist George S. Robertson, Ph.D., prove that the apple's bioactive compounds can significantly reduce oxidative stress and the risk of stroke.[7]

Furthermore, tests by research scientist H. P. Vasantha Rupasinghe, Ph.D., have shown that the darker side of an apple, where it absorbed the most sunlight, contains more nutrients than the less colorful side of the same apple. He adds: "The apple skin is unique. It contains two- to six-fold more antioxidants. People peel apples to avoid pesticides, but they're missing out on the antioxidants that are found specifically in the skin, not in the flesh."[8] This is yet another reason to choose organic produce—you don't have to peel it because it's pesticide free. To receive the most antioxidants, he recommends buying smaller apples. After all, two small apples have more skin than a large one.

In addition, red flower essences are reportedly good for the heart, blood circulation, energy, and vitality. In herbalism, red plants are used to treat fever. And pink and red are associated with the endocrine system.

Orange. Orange flower remedies are used to increase sociability, which is a characteristic of the second chakra.

Yellow. Yellow foods are associated with digestion ("yellow belly"), the solar plexus, the lymph system, cells, intestines, and the liver. In Chinese medicine, this color is associated with the stomach and spleen, and in Western herbalism, an olive (yellow green) color is associated with bile, which is a crucial part of the digestive system.

To get your energy moving first thing in the morning, drink some warm lemon water and tap on your kidneys, which are located near the spine at the small of the back. You can also add a little cayenne pepper as a wake-up call.

Look at how Nature's yellows are related to the stomach area. Ginger relieves upset stomachs and encourages bile flow. The bromelain in pineapple helps with digestion. Chamomile helps inflammation in the gastrointestinal tract.

Yellow flower remedies are often used for liver and self-esteem issues. Dark yellow flowers stimulate life force and the liver, while light yellow flowers help with internal cleansing.

Like Attracts Like

The root of the bright yellow dandelion has been proven to help the liver and gallbladder, and is associated with the third chakra. Dandelion's bitter taste gives us a clue that it will stimulate digestion. Its frayed leaves symbolize its ability to calm our nerves when we're feeling frayed. The leaves contain nerve-soothing niacin, as well as magnesium, potassium, zinc, and vitamin C complex. The fact that it's a sturdy plant shows that it can be a strong remedy for the body.

Green. Green plants store the energy they receive from the sun, and that energy becomes a part of the food you eat. Dark green plants are generally high in minerals and help the circulatory system. Cucumbers and fresh green juices are great for alkalizing your body, contributing to optimum health. (You'll get great results juicing fresh greens for a few days. You'll actually feel more energy; develop clearer, more vibrant skin; and gain new perspectives more easily.) Green foods also contain the micronutrient sulforaphane, which helps prevent cancer.[9]

Blue. According to author and berry researcher Paul Gross, Ph.D., dark blue, purple, or black fruits that easily stain your fingers during picking are great sources of anthocyanins, plant pigments that have numerous health benefits. Among other benefits, anthocyanins help eyesight and the nervous system, and they fight atherosclerosis.[10]

And interestingly, using small-sized sky blue plates may help you eat more slowly, because this light color has a calming effect on the brain. Dark blue fends off a large appetite.

Purple. Generally, purple flowers calm and relax you. This is no surprise because purple, the color of the seventh chakra, is known to be soothing and is related to spirituality in many cultures. Even Leonardo da Vinci believed that the power of meditating was up to ten times greater under a stained-glass window's violet light in a church.[11]

Black. According to Chinese medicine, black herbs and foods (such as nori, black rice, black cherries, black mushrooms, and black beans) help improve kidney function.

Color Therapy

"Color is the profound language of the soul, which needs to be learned like any other language. When the eye catches the visual vibration of color, it affects every cell of the body,"[12] explains Leslie Sloane, who has been a color therapist for 17 years and is the founder of Auracle's Colour Therapy. She is able to make uncanny, precise interpretations of what's going on in your psyche and health by simply looking at your color choices.

For example, when I first met her, in two minutes she looked at me and summed up that the right side of my thyroid was acting up. I had just visited my doctor who told me the exact same thing, but he charged me $1,200 and took up hours of my time.

Leslie says that generally people will choose or wear the color (or colors) that represents their consciousness since color *is* consciousness. In other words, colors are a message of the soul because we are made of light, and the full spectrum of the rainbow is held within the light. Therefore, all colors are contained in each cell of our bodies.

Colors are a language that most of us can't interpret just yet. We react to certain colors as we're going through different processes in our lives. Colors may speak of where we are off balance (physically, mentally, emotionally, or spiritually); what our desires are; what gifts we bring into this world to help humanity; and what our state of mind is (if we're depressed, we may be wearing blue often, and if we're filled with joy and laughter, we may be wearing lots of yellow). Leslie states: "Colors can tell of troubles in a relationship, whether someone is going through a transition in his or her life, and even speak of dis-ease. They will ultimately reveal where we are in harmony and where we are in discord."[12]

Color is all around us, and we react to it subconsciously. For instance, pink has a certain feel to it and can evoke a specific response. Depending on the circumstances, it might align us to a sense of vulnerability, fragility, feminine energy, kindness, tenderness, or unconditional love. Pink also signifies maternal energy, flowers, the soft underbelly of animals, and newborn babies.

Ways to Work with Colors

- *Examine which colors are missing in your surroundings.* Look at your clothes, food, and home decor; and notice if there are certain colors you tend to choose most often and which ones are missing. Think about why you avoid some colors and are attracted to others. Work on embracing a wider spectrum of colors in your environment.

- *Buy one new colorful food each week.* If you do this experiment faithfully, after a year you will have tasted over 52 new foods!

Getting in Touch with Nature—Literally

Nature's textures aren't random; they're very purposeful. The slippery leaf will help water the plant, and the leaf that has a rough texture at the bottom of the forest can absorb water. How often have you noticed the texture of the bark of one tree versus another or the smooth feel of grass or water caressing your feet?

Best-selling author Dr. Wayne Dyer explains that his writing process is deeply connected to sensory impressions in Nature:

> My inspiration came from nature in the most beautiful way. Before beginning each new chapter in the book, I would drive 35 miles east of where I live on Maui and then hike over an incredible number of rocks and through trees for about two hours. There's a place where a 50-foot waterfall drops into a pool, surrounded by guava trees covered with guava fruit. Here I would stay right under the waterfall and just let the water cascade down on my head. In the hours I spent there, everything I needed for my next chapter would appear. I didn't have an outline or any organization—just a beautiful, blissful place in the rain forest. It was almost as if God wrapped his arms around me and said, "This is what you'll need for the next chapter. Just be at peace."
>
> After a couple of hours of being out there in nature and finding my own nature, I would come back and sit down to write and everything just flowed so easily and so beautifully.[13]

To receive more of this inspiration, think of how as a child you were open to seeing all the wonders around you. Stephen Buhner outlines an exercise in his book *The Lost Language of Plants*, in which you meet yourself as a child in your imagination and then go on a walk in Nature and see what your "child" notices and likes.[14] Here's a modified version of his exercise:

Nature—Your Inner Child's View

Find a comfortable place to sit where you feel safe and know you won't be disturbed, preferably in Nature.

Close your eyes and take some deep breaths. Fill up your lungs as if they were balloons. Fill them almost to the point of bursting. Hold each breath for a few seconds then . . . slowly . . . release the air. As you let out the air in your lungs, release any tension you feel and let it go out with your breath. Do this again . . . several times.

Sit and relax. Imagine the earth upon which you are sitting to be huge hands that are holding and supporting you. Take some deep breaths.

Then imagine yourself as a child. Ask this child to come and join you. In your imagination, watch what the child enjoys in Nature and see what the child sees. Feel free to visualize your inner child at various ages. Spend as much time as you wish with yourself as a child, and see what you can discover about yourself that you had forgotten, or perhaps what you never really knew!

"And those who were seen dancing were thought to be insane by those who could not hear the music."

— **Friedrich Nietzsche**

🍃 🍃 🍃   🍃 🍃 🍃

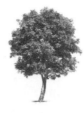

CHAPTER FIVE

- -

How Nature's Energy Boosts Your Energy

"Tell me what you eat and I will tell you what you are."

— **Anthelme Brillat-Savarin**

Nature's aliveness speaks to our life force. The more alive a food is, the more *chi* it has, and the more it can benefit us.

The electrical, vital energy of the food you eat is more important than how many calories it has. I've never known a radiantly healthy person who counted calories. Also, counting calories keeps you in your head rather than tuned in to the innate wisdom of what your body wants.

Going Beyond Nutrition

Let's travel far away from our multibillion-dollar diet industry to the rain forests where Nature keeps her bounty of secrets—hidden in plain sight.

Troy Casey, who attributes his recovery from alcoholism to Amazonian plants and herbs, claims that he searched the planet to find true healing at the core level and discovered that everything we need is in the rain forest. At 43 years old, he says that people often tell him how young and vibrant he looks, even though he has smoked for more than 20 years and used drugs and drank heavily for more than 10: "The plants of the Amazon have helped me restore my physical body, as well as my consciousness and spiritual connection to the Earth." He adds: "God doesn't make mistakes and did not leave us hanging without the ability to heal ourselves."[1]

The rain forest is appropriately called the "lungs of the planet," since its more than 200,000 species of plants help produce oxygen for the planet.[2] Notice how our lungs, with their alveoli (final branchings of the respiratory tree where the exchange of oxygen and carbon dioxide takes place), actually look like trees and keep the body's cells supplied with oxygen.

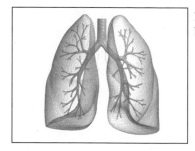

Note how our lungs actually mirror tree branches and both breathe life.

And here's another gift from Nature: the homeopathic remedy Spongia Tosta is made from dried and roasted sea sponges. It resembles the shape of the alveoli of the human lungs and is an effective treatment for a dry cough (without mucus or fluid).[3] You can purchase all-natural Spongia Tosta pellets online or at a health-food store.

An enormous amount of wisdom is packed into these dense natural areas of the planet. The Amazon's "superfoods" and herbs, which are rich in antioxidants and nutrients, far surpass most of our foods in nutritional value as well as in providing vital life energy. The rain forest's CamuCamu plant is an excellent example.

Nature's Secret Message
Diversity is the key to Nature's strength- and health-giving properties.

CamuCamu's Rich Diversity

The CamuCamu plant grows on the floodplain, where the water level rises 30 feet during the rainy season. That means that these plants are underwater for about three months. You'd think that they'd die, but they actually thrive there. Fallen leaves and other organic matter surround the submerged plants, adding nutrients, so that when the water recedes and the plants begin to reemerge, they're stronger and richer than ever before.[4]

The Amazon natives harvest CamuCamu and dry it, grinding it into a powder. Scientists are now finding that this plant creates a biological terrain in the brain that facilitates the uptake of serotonin, shifting our mind-set away from depression and toward optimism and joy. It also has anti-inflammatory and immune-enhancing properties, and even contains a full panel of B vitamins and certain amino acids that are essential for a balanced mood.

John Easterling, the founder of the Amazon Herb Company, explains that these plants are hardy because they're in a "survival of the fittest" environment in which only the strongest plants survive among the myriad species. He contrasts this to monocultural corn in Iowa that's grown in soil so lacking in biodiversity that the corn wouldn't naturally grow without the use of toxic chemicals. And it's also exposed to more pollutants from interstate highways toxins that the plants absorb.[4]

Nature's Secret Message
The quality and life force that a food contains makes a vast difference in your health.

When we eat foods grown in the rain forest, we're consuming their entire life-force experience. Rain-forest plants growing in mineral-rich soil contain energetic information about ecological balance and harmony that's approximately 100,000 years old. This is transferred to us when we eat the plants. Therefore, those of us who eat foods from the rain forest may feel more balanced and at peace because we're ingesting the plants' life-force energy.

Many people who struggle with obesity are actually lacking nutritionally, but those who eat dense, nutrient-rich foods feel more satisfied and function better overall. In fact, as Easterling contends: "You're introducing information into your body that's giving you a different and more conscious view of the world."[4] Could there be an energetic imprint of the plants that improves body function? Perhaps mass biodiversity can also be imprinted on the plant's cells.

We do know that food can affect us energetically by transferring its vitality to us and also by influencing the functioning of our chakras, as the blueberry seems to do.

Got the Blues? Eat Blueberries!

"Food governs your destiny."
— **Namboku Mizuno**

When we feel melancholy, we often say we have "the blues." So it's interesting to note that studies show blueberries, which are actually indigo (bluish purple), are proven to help with depression.

On the other hand, consider what's on the opposite side of the color wheel from bluish purple: yellow gold. We're referring to this hue when we speak of having a "sunny disposition" or a "golden opportunity." And wouldn't you know that sunflower seeds can lessen symptoms of depression because they contain the amino acid tryptophan, which is responsible for processing serotonin (the neurotransmitter that helps us feel good).

Another interesting observation is that the sunflower points upward and opens toward the sun, while the blueberry flower is closed and pointed downward. In fact, its droopy position makes it hard for bees to pollinate the flowers.

At this point, you've probably noticed what seems like an inconsistency here. If the happy-looking sunflower improves mood, why would the droopy little blueberry do the same? Remember, you have to observe many traits of the plant. Could its color be indicative of the energy centers in our bodies?

The blueberry's indigo color is the same color associated with the sixth chakra. (Chakras are widely regarded as invisible energy vortexes in the body.) The sixth chakra is universally associated with communication, meditation, and intuition. Check out the similarities between the blueberry and the sixth chakra:

Blueberries	Sixth Chakra
Are dark blue/indigo in color	Associated with the color indigo
Known as "brain berries," because they decrease oxidative stress to the brain[5]	Located on the forehead; symbolizes wisdom and intellect
Contain lutein, which delays eye problems associated with aging, with no negative side effects[6]	Represents vision and perception
Have shallow roots and no hairs or rootlets that reach into the earth	Related to the energy of the heavens—not the earth

Maybe all of the colors, shapes, and seeming inconsistencies are Nature's design so that everyone will be able to recognize what they most need to see at a particular moment. Like the well-known inkblot tests used by psychologists, there's no one right answer—there are just different interpretations that are appropriate for different people.

Nature's Secret Message
**Nature speaks to us through colors,
growth patterns, and shapes.**

Tips for Picking and Storing Blueberries

Remember to shake, rattle, and roll!

- If you pick up the container and the blueberries move around, that means they're fresh. If they're soft, damaged, or moldy, there *won't* be a whole lotta "rattling and rolling" goin' on!

- If you pick up a frozen bag and they're all stuck together, this could indicate that the berries have been thawed and refrozen.

"Power Plant" Presentations

Just as Microsoft's PowerPoint software creates dynamite presentations, Nature also constructs engaging power-*plant* presentations to intrigue her outdoor audiences! One example is mistletoe. This plant doesn't obey the rules; by the way it grows and behaves, it shows us that it addresses *imbalances*. For example, it can be used to treat cancer, an imbalance in the body.

Let's take a look at how this shrub stands out in Nature. Generally, a typical plant has roots in the ground; grows upward, toward the light; produces fruit or flowers during warm seasons; changes leaf color in the fall; and doesn't attach itself to sap trees. Mistletoe, however, doesn't have roots in the ground; rather, it grows in a ball shape on a tree. It doesn't depend on light; it's a parasitic plant that pulls nutrients from its host. In the winter, its leaves stay green, and it produces bright red berries.

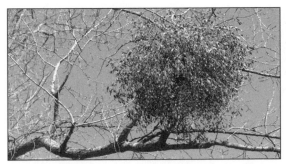

"Rebel with a cause." Mistletoe doesn't obey plant-kingdom rules (much like cancer cells, which also act abnormally), and is used as a treatment for cancer.

Mistletoe acts out of line with the rest of Nature! Philosopher Rudolf Steiner, the founder of the forward-thinking Waldorf Education system, observed the similarities between mistletoe growing on trees and the spread of cancer in the human body. How did Steiner discern this? Perhaps he looked at the plant's messages, hidden in plain sight.

"In health, it is asserted, the growth and organizing forces are operating in balanced harmony," Steiner said. "In cancer, however, the organizing processes, which are closely related to quality of individuality, personal uniqueness, are weak, and the growth process has gone out of control. What is needed is a strengthening of the individuality of the patient, of the formative forces that are concerned with control, order and independence. These, of course, are precisely the qualities that the mistletoe seems to exhibit in its independence from terrestrial and cosmic influences."[7]

Mistletoe	Cancer Cells
Doesn't obey many plant-kingdom rules	Don't obey signals from other cells
Looks abnormal (has a messy, misshapen form)	Look abnormal (form may be misshapen)
Grows on unhealthy trees	May grow in unhealthy bodies

Mistletoe is the "I did it my way" plant with its atypical rhythms, but is it exhibiting these unusual behaviors for a reason? Scientific studies show that mistletoe, marketed under the name

Iscador, is an alternative treatment for cancer. Suzanne Somers publicized this when she elected to use it to treat her breast cancer, as it has been extensively studied in Europe as a complementary treatment for tumors.

A study conducted in Germany and Switzerland involved 686 patients (329 on mistletoe and 357 controls) from 35 centers, who were observed for an average of 30 months. The results? "A significantly longer tumor-related survival was found in the FME [mistletoe] group when compared with the untreated controls," as stated in an article published in the journal *Alternative Therapies in Health and Medicine*. Researchers at Germany's Institute of Preventative Medicine concluded that Iscador can extend a cancer patient's survival time.[8] (**Note:** The use of Iscador, and other forms of mistletoe for medicinal use, is not a cure for cancer, but it has been used with other therapies to help in the treatment of cancer.)

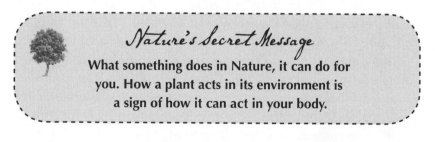

Nature's Secret Message
What something does in Nature, it can do for you. How a plant acts in its environment is a sign of how it can act in your body.

Knowing the unique traits of mistletoe may cause you to view this plant in new ways. Let's also look at the willow tree from a fresh perspective and try to learn what its power-plant presentation has to tell us.

What Weeping Willows Show Us

One day many years ago after a severe storm, my family and I found our small weeping willow lying on the edge of the lake in our backyard, attached to its roots only by a bit of bark on one side of the trunk. I wondered if it would survive Nature's powerful blow.

Determined to give it new life, my parents tenderly picked it up, wrapped it with tree tape, and staked it. As the tree willingly knit itself together, it eventually became strong enough to once again stand on its own, and the tape and stakes were no longer needed. What had appeared to be a loss was actually a rebirth.

Today I can no longer wrap my arms around its thick, sturdy, indomitable trunk! Is it nostalgia, or is there a deeper message in this magnificent tree? Can we, like the weeping willow, grow strong once again and find new life after weathering our own great storms?

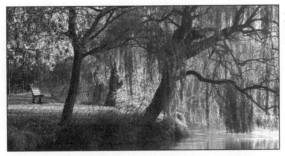

Aspirin was discovered by observing characteristics of the willow tree.

Throughout the ages, the willow tree's narrow, tear-shaped leaves and drooping branches have symbolized sadness. Yet its wispy branches and bitter bark suggest other emotions, such as pliability, tenacity, and resilience.

In the fall, I noticed another trait of the willow. It was the last tree to finally let go of its leaves, some of which were still clinging together as they made their journey to the ground. It reminded me that with all things, there's a time to let go. By hanging on to pain and sorrow, we're struggling against Nature, missing the possibilities of renewed strength that come with letting go and releasing what we no longer need.

The Wisdom of the Willow

Recognizing the qualities of the willow, Bach Flower Remedies and other essences capture the strength of this magnificent tree, helping us forgive past injustices and release resentment and bitterness. Likewise, aspirin was discovered from observing the willow tree's characteristics. Its supple branches, resembling flexible human limbs, were one of the many signs that pointed to its capacity to relieve joint pain. Hippocrates instructed people to chew on willow leaves for pain relief; and he also made a powder from the bark and leaves to treat fever, headaches, and pain.

In the 1700s, Edmond Stone conducted the first recorded human trials of willow as a pain reliever, giving 50 patients a dose of powder made from willow bark. He had observed several signs in Nature that the willow might be good for this purpose, such as a bitter taste, which can be a sign of medicinal power, and damp conditions in which the trees grew, which he correlated to aches and pains caused by damp, cold weather.

By 1829, scientists isolated the salicin (salicylic acid in its pure state) in willow bark, the compound that provided pain relief. Unfortunately, salicylic acid was hard on the stomach and tasted very bitter. In 1897, this medicine was synthesized into acetylsalicylic acid, and in 1899 it was marketed as Aspirin® (then a trade name). In fact, many discoveries in medicine began with an observation about the appearance of a plant.

Leaves of Three, Let It Be

Poison ivy has a power-plant presentation, too. Here's something you'll be itching to know! Avoid the "ivy threes." If a plant has a cluster of three leaves, it could be either poison ivy or poison oak—so steer clear of it. Another clue to look for is that the pointed leaves of poison ivy are green in the summer but reddish in the spring and fall.

If you end up suffering from a dose of poison ivy, you'll be especially happy to hear that another of Nature's secret messages is in the jewelweed plant, which is used to treat poison ivy and actually resembles the rash that erupts on a person's skin.

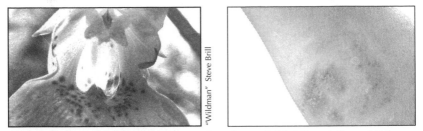

Notice the resemblance between a poison-ivy rash [right] and the reddish spots on the jewelweed plant [left] that's used to treat it.

Once again, what we're looking for is hidden in plain sight! Poison ivy shows us by its physical position (often right next to its antidote, the jewelweed or mugwort plants) that we can balance our energy *and* that the answers to our challenges are nearby. Our bodies work in a similar fashion, sometimes automatically knowing what to do when there's a problem. For example, if we ingest poison, we may vomit to remove the toxin from our system. If we feel chilled, we start to shiver in order to generate heat. In their amazing wisdom, the human body and Nature itself give us many clues *and* solutions at the same time!

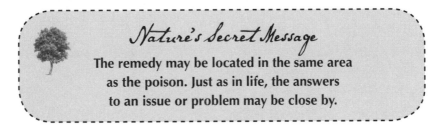

Nature's Secret Message

The remedy may be located in the same area as the poison. Just as in life, the answers to an issue or problem may be close by.

You can learn a great deal about yourself (and others) if you tune in to your senses and carefully observe all of the qualities of a living thing in the natural world. In Part II, you'll learn about Nature's lessons on emotions and the workings of your mind.

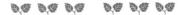

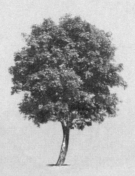

Part II

Nature's Secrets about Emotional
and Mental Well-Being

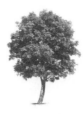

CHAPTER SIX

Water and Soil Mirror Our Bodies

*"Let the waters settle. You will see stars
and moon mirrored in your Being."*

— Rumi

Soil and water—two important elements of life on the planet—
have many lessons to teach us about our relationship to the natural
world. Too often, we let our emotions and thoughts dictate our
behaviors and perceptions instead of paying attention to Nature,
which serves as a healthy role model. Nature has many secret
messages to share with us on overloading and overstressing ourselves with toxicity, moving forward with fluidity and consistency,
remembering where our support lies, and respecting the earth that
nourishes us.

According to the research and educational organization Math/
Science Nucleus, ancient cultures considered water to be the essence
of life because it's vital to every organism on Earth. Throughout
time, rain was considered a gift of the gods from heaven; and even
today, many religions use holy water to cleanse the soul.[1] Before
we're born, we're submersed in water: a baby is surrounded and
cushioned by water in the womb. Like the ocean, our bodily fluids
are approximately 70 percent water; and our blood, sweat, urine,
and tears contain salt and are similar in composition to the sea.

Basic IV therapy (intravenous therapy), which is used in hospitals to nourish and hydrate patients, is a saline solution (salt water).

Let's compare some of the ways in which the human body mirrors this aspect of Nature:

Our Water World	Our Human Bodies of Water
Earth is approximately 70 percent water.	Our bodies are approximately 70 percent water.
The ocean is composed of salt water.	Body fluids (blood, sweat, tears, and urine) contain salt.
The sea contains approximately 90 minerals.[2] (These numbers are debatable.)	Our bodies contain approximately 92 naturally occurring elements known to play a role in normal function.[2] (These numbers are debatable.)
Stagnant conditions breed germs and bacteria, creating unhealthy water.	Stagnation in the body contributes to disease.

From Seawater to Seafood

Have you ever wondered which are the healthiest foods at the grocery store? If you guessed vegetables, you're only half right. Mineral-rich sea vegetables and seaweeds (such as nori, dulse, arame, and others) are excellent for your health, even containing up to ten times *more* nutrients than food grown on land. Notice how they mirror the fluids of the body, which are also packed with trace elements.

These sea veggies help low-functioning thyroids, a far-too-common medical issue in America. I've had personal experience with this: years ago, a top, super-expensive thyroid doctor informed me that I had to avoid iodine and that I absolutely needed thyroid medication. He then showed me pictures in medical textbooks of patients' grossly deformed necks that resulted from thyroid conditions.

I went home to do some research first. Days later, I called my doctor and requested an "iodine challenge test" to check my iodine levels. He snapped, "Why are you reading about this stuff? Stop reading! You're gonna get yourself in trouble." Since it's my body, I again requested the test, because I needed a prescription to urinate in a bucket (that's another story). My doctor finally wrote the prescription, but it was so illegible the lab had to call to verify what he'd written. Sure enough, when the test results came in, I discovered that I was very low in iodine. (Consider having your iodine levels measured, because replenishing iodine with sea veggies generally helps the thyroid. But if you have Hashimoto's disease or Graves' disease, iodine can worsen the thyroid. Check with your doctor to see what's best for you.)

I didn't take the strongly recommended thyroid medication, which would have required that I be on it for the rest of my life. It's been over six years since that visit to the thyroid doctor, and my neck doesn't look anything like the photos he showed me, and my health has also been very good. For me, the medication was not the right thing at the time, and I went the alternative route. However, this doesn't mean it would be the same for you because everyone is different. But I'm glad that I got other opinions and thoroughly investigated all my options before I made such an important decision that might require a lifetime of medication.

Iodine-rich sea veggies are great for your appearance, too. I recently saw a friend who looked more radiant than ever. When I asked what her secret was, she said that she's eating more sea veggies and replacing bread with nori sheets.

Is the thought of sitting down to a bowl of sea veggies unappealing to you? Well, there are many other ways to enjoy this nutritious food, which comes in a variety of tastes. For example, you can wrap your veggies in nori sheets or add slivers of sea veggies to rice dishes or salads.

Sea-Veggie Healthy Salt

You can grind several sea vegetables to create a healthy salt. Chef Teton, the star and creator of the *Essential Cuisine* DVD series, shares her iodine and mineral-rich recipe:

1. Purchase one bag of any or all of the following: kelp, wild Atlantic kombu, alaria, dulse, laver, and nori. Make sure you buy organic sea veggies, which contain no chemicals or additives and are from clean, unpolluted waters.

2. Take a handful from each bag and place in a blender. Blend, stopping often to loosen mixture from the base of the blender. Grind sea veggies into tiny flakes, varied in size.

3. Transfer to a glass jar with a lid, and sprinkle your sea-veggie salt on almost everything you eat. This nutritious mixture will last indefinitely.[3]

A River of Tears

Have you ever noticed how much better you feel after a good cry? Have you ever watched another person become visibly calmer and more at peace as he or she emerges from a storm of tears? This is due to the emotional and chemical reactions that are taking place. When you weep because of sadness or frustration, your tears contain up to 24 percent protein and are believed to release excess stress hormones.

Some people take antidepressants so that they *don't* feel sadness and cry. Is this wise, though? Perhaps if they allow themselves to experience their pain as well as a cathartic cry, they would feel better. (Please note that I'm referring to normal "blues" here, not severe depression.)

Our bodies are like Nature in that both strive for balance. Crocodiles cry "crocodile tears," but this has nothing to do with sadness; they "cry" to rid their bodies of excess salt. And according to Michael Lennox, Ph.D., a Los Angeles–based psychologist and expert in dream interpretation, a rainstorm cleanses the air, nourishes the earth beneath our feet, and is the closest thing to human crying. If we allowed ourselves to cry at times, what might we cleanse in our own lives? How might we strengthen ourselves?

So why not go ahead . . . drain away your pent-up feelings and release a river of emotional tears. You'll feel better!

The Lessons of Water

Observe how even a gentle stream of water can, over time, carve through rock and break down the hardest stone. By reflecting on water's consistent, persistent, and flowing nature, you too can receive positive results when applying these principles to your life.

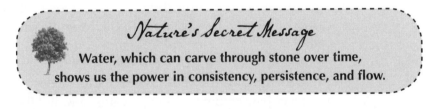

Nature's Secret Message

Water, which can carve through stone over time, shows us the power in consistency, persistence, and flow.

The internationally acclaimed singer Beyoncé is celebrated for her gorgeous figure. Her physical trainer, AJ Johnson, is often asked to divulge her client's fitness secrets. She answers in one word: *consistency.* It's not what Beyoncé does, explains AJ—it's the regularity that produces results. Doing any exercise once in a while doesn't produce results. I'm sure there are days that Beyoncé would rather sit on her famous booty and eat bonbons, but instead, she remains committed to her exercise program. It's similar to the Kundalini yoga teaching, "Keep up and you'll be kept up," which reflects the rewards of consistent action.

Water has an unstoppable nature, flowing over and around blockades, persevering as it moves forward. How can you be more like water—consistent, full of energy, flowing around and through obstacles?

"Only in quiet waters things mirror themselves undistorted. Only in a quiet mind is adequate perception of the world."

— **Hans Margolius**

The Waterfall Pose:
Imitating Water to Achieve Its Stress-Busting Benefits

The following exercises will allow more harmony and flow in your life. Here's why: stress puts you into a fight-or-flight response, which sends all your energy to your extremities (arms and legs) so that you can run from or defend against predators. Once you feel safe, the nervous system reverts to the rest-and-digest mode, with more blood flowing back to the rest of your body.

If you're constantly stressed, you stay stuck in the fight-or-flight reaction, which greatly upsets digestion. To bring your body back into relax-and-digest mode, you can trick it into thinking it's safe by encouraging more blood to flow into the digestive system, away from your extremities. Practically anyone can do this by taking a cue from Nature and assuming the restorative "waterfall pose." Simply elevate your legs by propping them up against a wall. Like water flowing downhill, your body's energy will move back toward the digestive organs.

Yoga therapist Colleen Carroll, founder of Sound Yoga Studio in Topanga, California, explains how this simple, effective yoga pose mimics Nature: "When the rivers of the earth change course, they purge and cleanse the ecosystem, and new life-forms appear. So, too, in the body, inversions are desirable for purification, release of stagnant energy, and change."[4]

If you find it difficult to prop your legs straight up against the wall, you can lie on the floor and place your legs on a chair or bed (see the following photos). Either way, you want to get the blood to flow back down to the stomach. Stay in this relaxing pose for 15 minutes, or longer if you wish. While you're in this pose, it's important not to chant, think too hard about anything, or listen to music—do nothing but relax. It's called "rest and digest" for a reason! It's also a good idea to use a rolled-up towel to support the back of your neck.

If you do this pose twice a day, you'll see an improvement in your digestion and overall health, and you'll also feel less emotional stress.

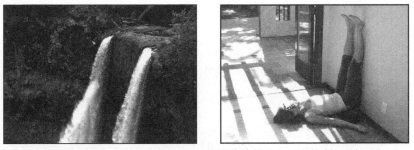

Model: Yoga Teacher: Holi Rabishaw
Photo Credit: Marcia Perel

By mirroring Nature, you can assume the "waterfall pose" [left] and trick your body into rest-and-digest mode.

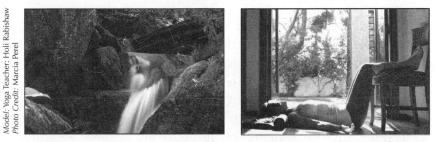

Model: Yoga Teacher: Holi Rabishaw
Photo Credit: Marcia Perel

The alternative "waterfall pose" [left] also mirrors Nature and creates the same stress-reducing benefits.

Nature's Secret Message
We, like Nature, need energy and movement to be healthy.

In Nature, fresh-flowing water can be likened to the healthy circulation of our blood. In contrast, stagnation reflects a lack of movement. Stagnant water can harbor bacteria and parasites and becomes a breeding ground for mosquitoes. Chinese medicine teaches that stagnant or blocked energy causes many health issues.

In what ways are you emotionally or mentally stagnant, unwilling to move? Healthy energy, like a running brook, is free-flowing, cleansing, and flexible.

The following exercise really helps to increase circulation. It's one of my favorites because anyone can do it just about anywhere, and it's free. Providing that you don't have any skeletal issues, *gently* bounce up and down from your knees, while keeping your feet on the floor. You can also gently shake your hands, arms, and legs; or wiggle your body to help the bodily fluids move more freely, like water flowing in Nature.

If you wish to achieve an even deeper state of relaxation, you can adopt the bathing rituals of the ancients, who knew the therapeutic secrets of water.

Baths:
Returning to the Source

In ancient Rome, bathing was a daily, communal activity. Throughout the world, "taking the waters" is known to be healing and rejuvenating. Religious pilgrimages have been made to places such as Lourdes, France, that are known for their healing waters. Even Hippocrates, the father of modern medicine, noticed that the cuts on a fisherman's hands healed faster with seawater, and he used it with other patients for pain relief and healing. Scientific studies now prove that Hippocrates (as with so many of his other techniques) was correct.

Numerous forms of water therapies exist. I went to the city of Baden-Baden (the name means "to bathe") in Germany to experience their world-renowned baths. I felt like one of the characters from *The Wizard of Oz* when they were "fluffed and buffed" before seeing the wizard. A large German Frau brushed my body with special dry-skin brushes until my skin looked sunburned. Then I was dipped in hot and cool mineral baths, hosed off, and finally swaddled in warm mineral-water-soaked sheets with only my face peeking out. I slept so soundly that when I woke up, I wasn't sure of the time, day, or year! All I knew was that I felt and looked like a brand-new shiny penny. The nurturing waters from the baths were marvelously rejuvenating.

Does relaxing in the bath somehow remind us of the safe oasis of contentment that we experienced in the internal ocean on the nine-month journey to birth? Perhaps this is what we sense when we float peacefully in a body of water, soaking in a tub or drifting downstream in a boat, raft, or inner tube.

Humans throughout time have engaged in various water therapies because there's tremendous healing power in water. When unable to be in the sea, bathing in water and mineral-rich bath salts is a refreshing way to feel more connected to Nature (because our bodies are mostly made up of water). The more connected and aware we become, the more we feel one with Nature again. Bathing is good for us physically, emotionally, and mentally because it takes us back "home."

Water also feeds our rhythmic cellular memory. A mineral-salt bath can help wash away stress and tension, muscle aches, and joint pain. It can also improve sleep, help internal circulation, soften the skin, alleviate water retention, and promote calm and inner well-being. The list of its healing properties, long known to the ancients, is endless. No wonder people throughout the world have established sacred bathing rituals.

You can create your own relaxing bathing ritual. When filling the tub, soak in positive intentions with these suggestions:

- Use salts containing minerals, with no chemicals, artificial colors, or perfumes. Adding natural fragrances or essential oils may also promote relaxation.

- Install a filter on your tub's faucet for cleaner, purer water.

- Keep a glass of drinking water nearby so you can rehydrate from the inside out, as well as from the outside in.

- Cleanse your skin with a salt scrub or loofah to make it feel especially soft and smooth.

- Give reflexology (the science of energy meridians) a whirl. Reflexologists claim that massaging the feet is comparable to massaging the entire body. Footbaths are also a great way to de-stress (and they use less water than filling up a whole tub).

Some people hesitate to take a bath for environmental reasons, especially when the region where they live is experiencing a water shortage. Enrico Melson, M.D., a Harvard- and Stanford-trained doctor, responds to this by saying, "Just bathe consciously, remembering that the water is a gift from the earth and must be respected. You might also consider filling the tub only partway or taking a sponge bath."[5] (You can read about additional ways to conserve water in the appendices at the end of the book.) If you're nearby a natural body of water, visit it often and, if you can, immerse yourself in it to experience its natural feel-good effects. Understanding the secrets of the flow, consistency, power, and gentleness of water may help you recognize those qualities in yourself. Remember that even in the womb you were nourished and supported by water.

> *Nature's Secret Message*
> **We were caressed by water in the womb, which is why we feel so at home in it and nourished by it.**

Although many of us do recognize our natural connection to water, we don't often think that we could also be intricately connected to *dirt*. However, soil is of great importance to our health and well-being.

Laying the Groundwork

> *"Malnutrition begins with the soil."*
>
> — **Peter Tompkins** and **Christopher Bird**

Dirt may not seem like a scintillating discussion topic. After all, it's certainly not a cocktail-party icebreaker. (Well, not this kind of dirt!) Most people rarely give it a second thought, except to stomp it off their shoes. Yet many scientists believe that our lives depend on the health of the soil. Healthy soil equals healthy people; therefore, unhealthy soil equals unhealthy people. Landscape designer and architect Lawrence Ziese of Ashcrow Landscape Design in Los Angeles offers an analogy: "The amount of microscopic living things in a handful of soil equals the sum of every human being ever born on our earth's history." There's a lot of ground to cover here!

The soil is a living organism, just like us—*really!* World-renowned soil scientist Albert Schatz, Ph.D., likens the soil to the human body: both need and use water, minerals, and oxygen to function. The following chart will help you understand the complexity of soil and how similar it is to our bodies.

The Soil	The Human Body
Needs minerals and trace minerals	Needs minerals and trace minerals
Needs water	Needs water
Needs oxygen	Needs oxygen
Contains microbes, which act like the cells of the soil	Composed of cells
Contains several million micro-organisms per teaspoon	Contains 25 million red blood cells per teaspoon
Can be healthy or "sick"[6]	Can be healthy or sick
Has delicate ecosystem interactions	Has delicate ecosystem interactions

"Dirty" Secrets

In the words of raw foods pioneer M. Bircher-Benner, M.D., from his book *Fruit Dishes and Raw Vegetables:* "Nutrition is not the highest thing in life. But it is the soil on which the highest things can either perish or flourish." Most of the food we eat is touched by what's in the soil. Unhealthy soil leads to unhealthy bodies, teaching us that we have to respect and take care of the ground beneath us, our foundation and home, so that it can take care of us. This interdependent, harmonious interaction is like a dance team, with Mother Nature as the farmer's partner. By responding to her every seasonal move, farmers today can follow the footsteps of ancient people, mindfully observing Nature's signs and cycles, instinctively communing with her and feeling the pulse of the land. Farmers traditionally planted only when Nature gave them the go-ahead, and they weren't motivated to push Nature into their own schedules to make a greater profit.

Ancient astronomers studied the angles, dates, and positions of the planets, stars, and sun; and they related their findings to fertility, plant-growth cycles, tides, and the seasons. This information is still used in biodynamic farming to benefit the soil.

Ehrenfried Pfeiffer, Ph.D., the author of *Bio-dynamic Farming and Gardening,* compares today's soil to an overburdened, overloaded machine. It can no longer endure the deluge of chemicals and unnatural growth forced upon it. Mother Nature's soil is not only stressed but it also hasn't been given time to renew itself. After giving "birth" to a field of crops, the earth needs to rest and regenerate—not be forced to continually keep producing.

Even the Bible, in Exodus 23, stresses moderation and rest:

> For six years you shall sow your land and gather in its yield, but the seventh year you shall let it rest and lie fallow, that the poor of your people may eat; and what they leave the beasts of the field may eat. You shall do likewise with your vineyard, and with your olive orchard.

Stressed soil that has been overfarmed and poisoned by chemicals produces nutritionally inferior crops. Similarly, when we allow ourselves to become overly stressed by physical, emotional, and mental toxins, we push ourselves too hard; and then we dramatically decrease our productivity and ability to create. Although agribusiness dominates our produce production, the green movement is creating a swing toward sustainable farming practices. Our soil may have a chance to recuperate.

The Power of Mud

People have used mud in external treatments for thousands of years. In 400 B.C., Hippocrates routinely slathered wet mud and clay over his patients' bodies, believing that disease existed where the mud dried first. This was amazingly smart thinking, as the body generates more heat where there's inflammation and disease, causing the mud to dry faster. Now we know this to be accurate, and modern noninvasive thermograms use heat distribution to detect breast cancer and other diseases.

Numerous studies prove the restorative powers of specialized mud treatments, which have been used in spas around the world. Throughout history, people have applied therapeutic mud to alleviate pain, detoxify the body, beautify the skin, and yield a sense of vibrancy and rejuvenation. Clinical nutritionists Lisa Klinker and Vicki Nevarde, of Dynamic Health Associates based in San Diego, use a special "mud" consisting of earth substances from around the world, including peat, volcanic clay, and various minerals. They claim that their therapeutic mud acts like a magnet, pulling toxins out of the skin and reestablishing proper energy flow and vibrancy. When I used it as a facial mask, my skin felt noticeably smoother. In fact, afterward, I looked like I had makeup on! I now use mud masks often and really like the smooth feeling they give my skin.

However, we overwhelm the soil when we dump large amounts of toxins, particularly inorganic ones, onto the ground. Likewise, are there times when we overload our bodies, minds, and hearts with wasteful materials, not allowing ourselves time to process it into something of value? By respecting the soil and its need for time to "digest," we learn that we, too, must not overwhelm ourselves with physical, emotional, and mental stress.

The Earth's Heartbeat

We rarely think of the soil as having an energetic force, but it certainly does. Here's a secret for reaping its benefits for free: *Just touch Mother Earth!* Create harmony in your life by literally connecting with Nature, especially if you spend a lot of time in cities, walking in shoes on concrete, working in skyscrapers, and driving in cars.

Studies show that the body's cells respond to the earth's core frequency, known as the "Schumann Resonance." Sleep and magnetic-field expert Paul Becker, inventor of EarthPulse™ Geomagnetic Field Supplementation, said that Schumann waves (natural frequencies of the earth, sometimes referred to as the Earth's heartbeat) have conditioned our evolution. These frequencies particularly affect the healthy balance of our brain state and the energy in all the cells' mitochondria (which turn nutrients into energy, acting like tiny power plants). In other words, the Earth's "geopathic vitamins" are a recipe for harmony in the body.

These natural waves or frequencies are well under 20 beats per second, compared with the 50 to 60 cycles per second that power nearly everything related to modern life, including cell-phone and telecommunication networks. Becker adds that in today's environment, it's nearly impossible to receive this natural "tuning," as these emanations are drowned out by man-made higher frequency fields.[7]

NASA created a Schumann-wave stimulator (a magnetic-pulse generator mimicking the earth's frequency) after noticing how astronauts' physical condition severely deteriorated while they were in space, away from Earth's Schumann Resonance. This device gives them a steady supply of Earth energy.

The only other way to get back in touch with "Earth energy" is by camping beyond the grid of modern electric and telecommunication networks. The reason why you sleep so well when you're in a natural environment isn't due to the fresh air and exercise so much as the fact that you're sleeping in contact with the ground, in an environment that lacks most of the man-made electric and magnetic fields.

Nature's Secret Message

The earth's ground, dirt, grass, water, and sand can help ground you, putting you in touch with its nurturing energy and natural frequencies.

Getting Grounded

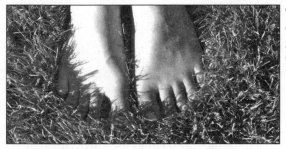

The earth's powerful energies can literally ground you and can even relieve symptoms of jet lag.

Nature is far more multifaceted than we realize, and its health is directly related to our health. Its vitality supports our vitality. The life in the soil and the ground's energy can . . . well, ground you. It can also make you feel centered, calm, and revived. If you're feeling stressed out, take off your shoes and walk on the grass or anywhere on a natural surface. You can feel a similar effect by being immersed in the ocean.

Maoshing Ni, Ph.D., the best-selling author and expert in Taoist anti-aging medicine, has a recommendation for alleviating jet lag—a manifestation of not being "grounded." When you arrive at your destination, he suggests, stand barefoot or lie down on the soil or grass to draw the earth's energy into your body. Putting your feet or body on the soil or grass (or in a river or ocean) gives you a free dose of the planet's good-feeling "vibes." If you can, also get some sunshine and drink plenty of water.[8]

Feeling the Earth's Support

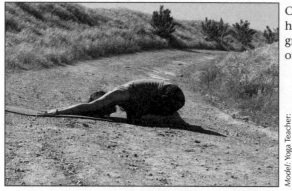

Child's pose [pictured] helps you feel the grounding support of the earth.

Model: Yoga Teacher: Holi Rabishaw, Photo Credit: Marcia Perel

The following exercise uses the earth's energy to calm you down and help you feel supported when you're feeling stressed. Kneel and bend forward, placing your forehead to the ground. In yoga, this posture is called the "child's pose." As you hold this position, imagine negative energy flowing out of you and into the earth from your third eye (the point between your eyebrows). If you find this pose difficult, you can simply lie on your stomach and visualize negative energy moving from your forehead into the ground. Simply feel the earth comfort you.

You can also lie with your solar plexus on the ground and visualize the ground supporting you, while all of the negative energy pours out of your body and into the ground.

Letting the Earth Handle Your Stress

Many people, when worried or stressed, tend to live in their heads, losing the connection to their feet and legs, and to the earth. Johnny Seitz, the body physiology expert whom I introduced earlier in this book, recommends the following grounding technique:

It's best to do this exercise barefoot on the ground. Turn out your feet slightly; put all your weight on your right foot while pushing into the ground and holding your balance, feeling a solid connection with the earth. Imagine moving your energy into the ground. Mother Earth can easily take on and dissipate your stress. Then repeat using your left foot. Keep walking this way, firmly balancing on each leg, releasing the tension stored in different areas of your body.

"The human body is the universe in miniature. . . .
The universe within reflects the universe without.
It follows, therefore, that if our knowledge of our own
body could be perfect, we would know the universe."

— **Mahatma Gandhi**

❦ ❦ ❦   ❦ ❦ ❦

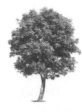

CHAPTER SEVEN

The Mind's Resistance to Nature's Genius

*"If the power to think is a remarkable gift,
the power not to think is even more so."*

— **Sri Aurobindo**

I got the phone call that everyone dreads—the one that starts with: "I went to the doctor . . ." Clouds numbed my mind as the hurricane of emotions approached. An MRI of my mother's shoulder revealed a 4.2 centimeter mass on her lungs and would require a CT scan for further evaluation.

My mom took the film to a pulmonary specialist who noted that the mass hadn't appeared on an x-ray taken only 11 months before then and quickly explained that a mass that large must be tested immediately. She continued on, explaining how cancer cells (*What cells?!*) double, then double again, and so on. This doctor had no idea what she was planting in my mother's mind.

She then handed my mom a referral for immediate PET and CT scans, with the "C word" etched on the paper. The word *cancer* stunned my mom, but the specialist continued her monologue, rapidly stating that a biopsy would come next, which would determine the type of treatment they'd start.

At this point, my mom was overloaded and overwhelmed, unable to grasp it all and reeling with memories of lung cancer in her family.

Her mind suddenly became the director of this act on the stage of her life, replacing the "stars" (her positive thoughts) with crowds of "extras" (fear, stress, and worry) who promptly took over the show.

In a fog, she heard the doctor say that she normally doesn't call anyone on the phone with bad news, but because of the long drive, she would save my mom the trip and call her when she received the results. Before leaving, she advised my mom, "Have someone with you when you get the call." *The* call. It was ominous.

I booked the next flight to Chicago. In the terminal, before my departure, a gentleman watched my unsuccessful attempts to make change for the pay phone and then graciously lent me his cell phone. After making my call, I returned his phone, but before the thanks could come out of my mouth, his face blurred as another silent flood of tears poured from my eyes. We sat in a cocoon of silence in the hubbub of the terminal, then we slowly began to speak about life. My vulnerability broke through all the superficialities—we simply connected. We were strangers sharing our lives with few, but meaningful, words, and I took some comfort from his compassion.

On the plane, I happened to sit next to a husband and wife who were researching new ways to deal with intense pain. I listened attentively to what they had to tell me, thinking their information might help my mom. As it turned out, the woman suffered from such excruciating pain that it would cause her to faint. She believed that her body was shutting down in order to cope with the unbearable pain. I marveled at the body's wisdom.

When I asked for her best tip on how to cope, she declared, "Think of something else! When you focus on pain, you get more of it." During her bouts of intense agony, she'd engross herself in a movie or have her husband read stories to take her mind somewhere else. She also meditated to keep her body focused and relaxed, and whenever her mind wandered, she would treat it like a precious puppy, lovingly coaxing, "Come back, sit, stay," as a gentle reminder.

She offered me another tip for meditating: stare into the middle of your forehead with your eyes closed; or with your eyes barely open, stare at the tip of your nose. Fixing your eyes on one spot really helps to still the mind. This woman now helps others manage their pain. She's taking her darkest hours and turning them into light for others.

The Wait

I arrived in Chicago to see my mom looking drained—she hadn't been sleeping. The doctor's blunt words kept racing through her mind, stuck on repeat. Waiting for the diagnosis seemed like an eternity. Time dragged as each . . . second . . . passed. The results were taking longer than usual because it happened to be during the holidays, and many offices and labs were closed.

Finally, the phone rang. It was *the* call. I handed the phone to my mom, and as she quietly listened to the doctor say, "Both tests show no signs of cancer," I saw years disappear from her face. I watched firsthand how words have as much power over the mind as disease. The "before" and "after" of my mom's appearance and attitude were astonishing—*all because of a few words!*

My point in sharing this story is to illustrate how we mirror Nature in that our thoughts (or even the words we hear) are seeds planted in the fertile soil of our mind. Those thoughts, when tended, eventually grow and bear fruit. But our mind (like the soil) will grow only what we plant in it. Flower seeds become flowers, not trees. Lemon trees produce lemons, not apples. We reap what we sow, both in Nature and in the garden of our mind. *So be careful what you plant!*

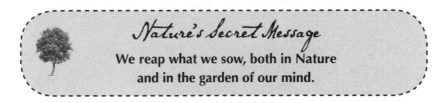

Nature's Secret Message
**We reap what we sow, both in Nature
and in the garden of our mind.**

In addition, weeds can run amok and take over the garden if you don't pull them out. In the same way, your "weeds" of worry and fear can choke the healthy seeds in your mind. Why not view

93

your problems as the earthworms that aerate and help drain the soil, actually working for your ultimate good?

Imagine your mind as a garden. What does it look like? Is it filled with beautiful flowers, and is it peaceful to walk through? What thoughts are producing those lovely buds? Do you see any weeds? If so, what's causing them to grow? What do you need to do to nurture the plants you want, and how can you remove the weeds that threaten to crowd out your beautiful flowers?

When we use the intangible fruits of our mind to help heal ourselves, can we actually trump Nature? I once read about a man who had chest pains and was sent for a chest x-ray. Unbeknownst to the man, his doctor died before he could call with the results. Somehow, the test results fell through the cracks, and not hearing otherwise, the man assumed that everything was okay and he was healthy. A few years went by, however, and he had another x-ray. This time his new doctor informed him that, judging by the x-ray, he had only a few months to live. A short time later, the man died. After his death, they compared his first x-ray to the second one and found that they were identical.

See how the body can obey the mind? What would happen if a team of doctors dropped in on a hospital patient and announced: "We were mistaken. You can go home now—you're fine!" Would that patient get better just by hearing those words? In the garden of our mind, words and thoughts are powerful seeds.

Mind Over Fatter

Karen Mangini is a 56-year-old "fit model" (or "fitting model") who's paid $125 an hour by designers to fit their clothes on her perfect size-6 body. She e-mailed me her secrets for maintaining her figure for more than 30 years.

Karen learned these longevity techniques from shamans of the Ecuadorian rain forest. Anyone can use these easy mental exercises to stay fit, healthy, and happy. The key is that she's learned to love her body—even its flaws! The method that Karen developed over the years is based on intuitive eating, self-love, and empowering thoughts. Her "mind over fatter" principles are as follows:

1. I never bought into the collective unconscious beliefs that our bodies change for the worse as we age. I listen to my body and project the positive feelings and images of health, vibrancy, and regeneration into my future.

2. I have an internally focused exercise program that succeeds in raising metabolism. I go to the gym once a week and imagine my muscles getting stronger and fuller, securing themselves firmly to the bone, and I hold that mind-set.

3. As I'm falling asleep, I imagine my entire body moving to a dance routine. My nerves, cells, muscles, and brain all respond as if I were actually dancing.

4. I have a positive, guilt-free attitude about and around food. I imagine my body easily digesting the nutrients and eliminating potential toxins. My secret is that I don't count calories—I count nutrition and enjoyment.[1]

Karen explains that if you don't believe that the mind can control the body, look at people who have a multiple personality disorder: with each "personality," their actions and behavior, and whether they feel pain or exhibit physical symptoms of a condition or illness, or even have allergies, can all change. In addition, studies show that basketball players who imagined shooting hoops in their mind scored almost as well as those who consistently practiced! Similarly, many golfers visualize where they want the ball to go before they take a swing. Can *you* imagine yourself successfully achieving your goals?

We've seen how the people around us and ourselves can influence our thoughts and beliefs. Now let's look at what we can learn from the ways in which Nature can impact an entire community.

Nature's Collective Mind:
The Amazing Wisdom of Bees

Bees know far more than we do about working together to sustain life. We often ignore Nature's wisdom and focus too much on how to help ourselves as individuals, which only creates even more emotional stress in our lives. Bees, on the other hand, share "hive intelligence" and serve the larger group instead of just themselves, ensuring everyone's survival.

These amazing creatures are known for their extraordinary teamwork and ability to work in harmony, even in tightly crowded spaces. Look at the following picture of the inside of a hive. Can you imagine humans getting along (and being productive) in those working conditions? What might bees know that we don't?

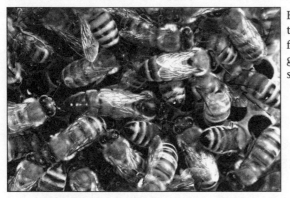

Busy bees work together in harmony for the good of the group. There's not a single "I" in bees!

Too often, we resist living cooperatively with others. We give in to fear and distrust and focus only on taking care of ourselves, which sets us up for loneliness and depression. We think, *If it's going to get done, it's up to me to make it happen*, and we overlook the importance of equality and community. What we could learn from the bees!

Bees are a prime example of how to productively live, work, and "be" together. And like the swarms of bees in Nature, there are also herds of elephants, schools of fish, packs of wolves, flocks of birds, colonies of ants, pods of dolphins, and so on . . . and they all work together within their groups. Humans are social beings as well. The individuals who most often commit crimes are loners; for example, shootings at schools are usually carried out by students who feel isolated from their classmates. Nature shows us the value of our participation in supportive communities.

> *Nature's Secret Message*
>
> **Generally, Nature's animals and insects are social.**

How can you create more positive relationships in your life? In his timeless classic *Think and Grow Rich,* Napoleon Hill attributes his success to a "Master Mind" group and defines it as: "The coordination of knowledge and effort, in a spirit of harmony, between two or more people, for the attainment of a definite purpose."[2] Could your own Master Mind group—a sort of think tank—support and help grow your intentions, your work, and/or your sense of community? Because everyone sees things differently, this type of gathering could offer you fresh perspectives, inspirations, and solutions. These groups can help put wind in your sails—much like geese flying in a V formation, flapping their wings to create a 71 percent greater lift for the birds behind them than if they flew alone. Master Mind groups can focus on any topic, take place in person or over the phone, and can include people from all over. (You can find suggestions on creating and maintaining harmonious, supportive Master Mind groups at the end of this chapter.)

Swarm Intelligence:
Instead of Thinking *Me*, Think *We*

One bee may not be so smart, but an entire hive is extraordinarily wise. Bees engage in what's called "swarm intelligence." (Other groups in Nature, such as ant colonies, exhibit this as well.) With as many as 50,000 bees in one hive, they make decisions, resolve conflicts, and do what's best for the whole, while still encouraging diversity and competition of ideas. We could learn from bees and start trusting that most people have much to offer us instead of being suspicious and cautious, closing ourselves off to others.

After researching the cooperative, successful decision-making behavior of honeybees, Cornell University biologist Thomas Seeley began modeling his faculty meetings on Nature's principles. For example, he asks all members of the group to express ideas and possibilities, and then they vote by secret ballot. Seeley states, "It's exactly what the swarm bees do, which gives a group time to let the best ideas emerge and win. People are usually quite amenable to that."[3]

"The bee is more honored than other animals, not because she labors, but because she labors for others."

— **Saint John Chrysostom**

Bees are great teachers: they exhibit generosity of spirit, sharing, and the importance of community. Guess what a bee does when it finds a new treasure of food? It doesn't hoard the prize for itself; it returns to the hive to share the good news via a "waggle dance," shaking its body in a manner that conveys information to the hive about the food's location. It's their version of MapQuest or a GPS!

How many humans would share their "treasure" for the benefit of others, to be in service to the group? Most feel that they already have too much to do, with pressures at work, a mortgage to pay, kids to feed, a home to run, and so on . . . however, like the spirit of the bees shows, service can be immensely fulfilling. Volunteers mention the benefits of service work, including feeling more grateful, uplifted, humbled, and profoundly connected with life, along with gaining rich, meaningful, rewarding experiences.

How to Apply the Lessons of the Bees
to Create Trustworthy and Inspiring Relationships

After writing a book about successful people (called *Outliers: The Story of Success*), Malcolm Gladwell sums up his theory: "No one . . . ever makes it alone." That's why Master Mind groups are helpful, because people receive support and gain fresh insights from each other.

Sometimes you can't see the forest for the trees, and this is where a Master Mind group would be effective. For instance, you may need help coming up with a name for your business or how to best market it (or you might need guidance with a weight-loss plan or some other personal goal), so you ask the group to start brainstorming. They can assist you with accountability, too. All members get a set amount of time to state their insights and opinions in a lighthearted, positive manner.

Here are some guidelines:

- Create a group where everyone is supportive, harmonious, and helpful. Emphasize win-win relationships.

- Help others by listening, thinking up new ideas, and flushing through the ones that are already being used. Avoid complaining, gossiping, defending, or playing the victim.

- Designate a specific amount of time for each person to speak uninterrupted on whatever topic he or she needs help with. (Twenty to thirty minutes should suffice.) *It's very important to stick to the agreed amount of time for each person.* When time is limited, people tend to focus better and accomplish more.

- Maintain a light and caring approach. A positive, fun atmosphere always generates fresh ideas. This isn't brain surgery—it's enjoyable brainstorming.

Mastermind with a Friend

You can also mastermind with a friend, with each of you taking from 5 to 30 minutes to focus on your topic. Remember to time it so the discussion stays focused. Leave "gab time" for another occasion. You can even share your goals for the day with a friend. There's something about speaking your intention to another person that gives it added power and clarity.

Mastermind with Your Imagination

Some students at Harvard Business School have been taught to create an imaginary Master Mind group. One student told me how he received remarkable clarity when he chose his heroes, living and dead, to meet every morning (in his mind) to go over his plans and offer advice.

Using this exercise, you have the opportunity to also ask anyone in the world, living or dead, what they would do in your situation. Go ahead, converse with a billionaire about your business plans, or ask a spiritual leader about your purpose. Ask away—there are no limits, and it's free! You may be surprised by the profound wisdom your mind conjures up.

🌿 🌿 🌿

Next let's take a look at what Nature can teach us about how she deals with time. Our frenzied attempts to squeeze more and more into every hour is very different from her rhythmic cycles. Could we improve the quality of our lives by simply mirroring Mother Nature's perception of time?

🌿 🌿 🌿   🌿 🌿 🌿

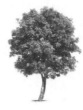

CHAPTER EIGHT

Nature's Time vs. Our Time

"Impatiently rushing produces no result."

— Chinese proverb

Late one night I was leaving a trendy Beverly Hills nightclub with my good friend Robin. As we strolled by an alley, I heard a scuffle behind us. I turned around and saw two men, one of whom was pointing a gun at me.

My mind couldn't make sense of this unexpected experience. *Was this a joke?!* Suddenly, time s-l-o-o-o-w-e-d w-a-a-a-y d-o-w-n. It was just like in the movies, when the actors are fleeing from danger and the film shifts into slow motion. At that speed, everything is sharp and clear. I saw every detail, and I can even remember the way the streetlight reflected off the shiny surface of the gun. In that moment, there was no time, no thought, no judgment—simply 100 percent pure attention. (Thankfully, Robin and I were unharmed! In a brave move, my friend threw her wallet far off and yelled at the miscreants to take the money and leave us alone.)

Similarly, I once heard a woman describe the fateful moment she became a paraplegic. She was climbing in a tree, high up in the branches, when she stepped on a dead limb. The moment the branch snapped, time slowed to a crawl and she felt like a feather, gently floating through the air, even noticing the sunlight streaming through the leaves. She had no thoughts or fears, despite the fact that she was falling. The event was seemingly timeless.

"For fast-acting relief, try slowing down."

— Lily Tomlin

Most of us live as if we're going 100 miles an hour. We're thinking about many things at once, and the majority of those thoughts have nothing to do with what's presently happening, but with something that will happen later on—like what we'll make for dinner that night, when we think we might get that promotion, what we should do for a loved one's birthday, or even how much we need to be saving for a child's college tuition or our own retirement. However, this is *not* the message we get from Nature about how best to stay in balance.

The ancients, for example, who based their ideas about time on Nature's rhythms, were sensitive to and in tune with the earth. The farmer of years past could feel the weather in his bones and would work from sunrise to sunset, planting in accordance with Nature's signs and also by observing the moon, sun, and stars. Our ancestors understood that we're a part of the natural world, and that the moon and planets and their cycles relate to the plants around us, and even to the organs in our bodies.

We have proof of this from one of the first "clocks," called the antikythera mechanism (an astronomical calculator), which was discovered in a shipwreck. Thorough examination of this ingenious device revealed that ancient Greeks could keep track of the time with calculations of the changing positions of stars and planets—almost like a computer. Professor Mike Edmunds of Cardiff University in Wales reveals: "This device [the antikythera] is just extraordinary, the only thing of its kind. The design is beautiful, the astronomy is exactly right."[1]

It's now très chic to employ biodynamic farming methods, which includes using only organic materials for fertilizing and soil conditioning. This is especially popular among the most celebrated vintners, who believe that an all-natural farming technique creates a better tasting, juicier grape, which in turn produces a finer wine. Learning from the ancients, they harvest according to certain lunar phases and observe how the fruit reacts to its environment instead of pushing it to harvest so that it fits into a specific time schedule. Biodynamic farming takes everything into account—not just our wants—and it also avoids the use of pesticides and chemicals, which have far-reaching effects.

And guess what the farmers report. According to an interview with Piero Incisa, who uses biodynamic techniques at his vineyard in Patagonia: "Since biodynamic methods were introduced at Chacra, the plants seem stronger, the leaves greener and the fruit more balanced, with better acidity." Incisa says, "The vineyard really isn't so different from a human being. If I don't do drugs or smoke, and I exercise, I'll feel better."[2]

Similarly, consider the ebb and flow of the tides. According to the Mayans, this pattern mirrors the times of the day when human energy is at a high or low. When the tide is low, they believed it was a time for rest; when the tide was high, it signified the time for productivity. Our bodies are designed to be in tune with Nature. How often do we resist fatigue or ignore the ebb and flow of our changing energy? According to Paul Nison, author of *The Daylight Diet,* even our body's digestion changes in line with Nature's cycles, which he expresses in his catchy rhyme: "When the sun goes down, digestion slows down. When the sun is out, digestion's best, no doubt."

Are your overbooked schedules with too much on your plate and crammed activities going against Nature's laws, putting you out of sync with Nature's time? We've developed a mental habit of racing against time. We try to bend time to our mind's needs and think that we must fit more hours into the day, so we live by artificial light. Our unnatural ideas blind us to the serenity of Nature's unhurried cycles.

Nature's Secret Message
Animals in Nature live in the moment without worrying about the future.

For example, our mind's ideas about food production and profit cause us to rush the maturing of the chickens we eat so that we can harvest their meat faster. We overlook the nutritional impact this might have and disregard whether being out of sync with Nature causes harm to the animals. What happens when we force Nature to change her timing? In 1960, it took baby chickens 11 weeks to reach maturity; in 2005, it took only 6 weeks. What's happening is that the chickens are growing too fast for their body, and their young legs can't support the rushed growth. This results in tissue damage and joint pain, and it prevents the birds from standing and walking—what they naturally need to do to be healthy and develop nutritious meat.

Just like the chickens, when we get too far away from Nature's timing, our bodies don't respond favorably. Studies show that sleep disturbances can result from not being exposed to the first morning light and spending the majority of our hours in artificial lighting.

We could choose to live more consciously and take our clues from Nature's wisdom. George Sobol, a Transcendental Meditation teacher for Maharishi Mahesh Yogi and teacher of Siddha Yoga for Swami Muktananda, recalls how he experienced transcending time ("beyond your mind, body, and emotions") in a surfing accident. He heard the bones in his neck cracking over the roar of the waves when his head hit the beach like a pile driver. He witnessed himself pray, *God help me!* This observation was from the perspective of his unbounded Self—the pure consciousness that we are—beyond time and space. He explains that this is a glimpse of the experience we can have permanently by utilizing techniques such as meditation to calm our mind and connect to our inner Truth—the all-pervading Intelligence that's always in harmony with Nature. This reminds him of the St. Francis quote: "That which you are looking for, is that which is looking."

We receive this peaceful calm when we slow down and live in Nature's timing.

"The Pace of Nature"

Are we ignoring the importance of the earth's timing and rhythm? Nothing is ever rushed, yet Mother Nature somehow manages to get everything done. The documentary *Play Again* reports that the average child recognizes more than a hundred corporate logos but can't name ten types of plants. I wonder that if this trend were reversed, would attention deficit disorder (ADD) be so alarmingly widespread?

Edward M. Hallowell, M.D., describes what it's like to live with ADD: "In ADD, time collapses. Time becomes a black hole. To the person with ADD it feels as if everything is happening all at once."[3] Interestingly Richard Louv, the author of the national bestseller *Last Child in the Woods: Saving Our Children from Nature-Deficit Disorder,* asserts that incidences of ADD and ADHD (attention-deficit/hyperactivity disorder) are lessened when children spend time in Nature. In fact, research conducted at the University of Illinois shows that children who had more "green time" exhibit a dramatic reduction in the symptoms of ADHD and ADD. Does Nature's rhythm relax people and reset their internal clock and mood?

Recall a day you spent outdoors. Didn't time seem to disappear? Lying on the grass, you looked up at the trees and saw the sun's rays pouring through the branches and the leaves dancing in the rhythm of the wind. The shape-shifting clouds became a variety of images on the canvas of your mind. You amused yourself with a trail of ants, traveling in a long row, and thought how much it was like a crowded freeway. And when you got up to go home, you felt rested and calm, yet awake, alive with energy.

One reason why people feel so serene after being outdoors is because of Mother Nature's timelessness. She doesn't keep appointments, schedules, alarm clocks, or to-do lists! She doesn't pressure the flowers to grow faster. Nature adheres to her own timing, and when we connect to her rhythm, we discover a sense of utter peacefulness. Ralph Waldo Emerson sums it up this way: "Adopt the pace of Nature. Her secret is patience."

Unfortunately, in today's society, it seems like our busy, busy lives are always speeding up, but what we need to do is slow down and take a "time-in."

How to Take a Time-In

You may find yourself thinking, *Yeah, yeah . . . I just don't have time for this! I have places to go, things to do now! I'm on a deadline! I've got to hurry!* Not only do you get out of sync with Nature's time, but you can also go so fast that you forget your purpose. Psychotherapist Len Worley, Ph.D., offers invaluable insights into how he stopped rushing around, and instead, befriended time:

> This is a spiritual practice for me, listening to how my body perceives. A dozen times a day or more, I check in with my body to see what it desires. What do I want to have for lunch? (A slight tension is felt if I'm choosing food that my body doesn't desire.) Should I say yes to the invitation to attend that concert next Wednesday? (My body feels an excitement and relaxed feeling, so I say yes.) I'm rushing to do just one more errand before making my next appointment—I listen to the tension and realize that I can do the chore later, and so I arrive on time and I'm more present for my next appointment.[4]

Worley shares the following practices for tuning in to natural guidance through feelings you experience in your body:

- *Trust tiredness.* Don't push your body with stimulants.

- *Nap often.* The mind can reestablish equilibrium and be far more creative when it's rested. Runners relax before races to increase stored energy in their muscles. A field that has rested produces beautiful crops.

- *Slow down.* Walk more slowly, whether you're going across the room, from your car to the grocery store, or down the street. Are you enjoying a stroll or rushing to get to that next appointment?

- *Talk with pauses.* Pay attention to how fast you're talking. Is there room between sentences? Between words?

- *Move with elegance.* Notice, for instance, how hectic or relaxed your hands are when washing the dishes.

- *Live with feeling.* The faster you go, the less you feel (other than anxiety).

- *Be sensual.* In every breath you take . . . how deep and full do you make it? Get in touch with the pleasure of breathing—not just during meditation, but all the time.

- *Write it down.* Take time to journal about what your life would be like if you didn't feel pressured by time.

- *Go outside.* Allow yourself to go outside and enjoy a natural setting. Can you go out in Nature this week and embrace its timelessness?

So the next time you feel yourself rushing around (or catch yourself worrying about some future event) instead of focusing on what's happening in the present moment, *take a breath*. Remember the wisdom of Nature, and take your cues from her timing. Identify the natural rhythms around you and within your own body, and strive to be in harmony with them. You'll soon see how much more smoothly and peacefully everything will go.

As you'll read in the next chapter, this more authentic rhythm will allow you to focus in a new way, and you'll be able to relax into a state of allowing abundance to flow freely and naturally to you. My guess is that you'll prefer that to the stressful battle of wills you may be currently used to!

"Nature's peace will flow into you as sunshine flows into trees. The winds will blow their own freshness into you, and the storms their energy, while cares will drop off like autumn leaves."

— **John Muir**

❧ ❧ ❧   ❧ ❧ ❧

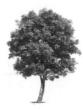

CHAPTER NINE

Nature's Winning Secrets

"Don't ask yourself what the world needs. Ask yourself what makes you come alive, and go do that, because what the world needs is people who have come alive."

— **Howard Thurman**

My whole body trembles as my sweaty hands pick up the dice. I throw them with so much nervous energy that they go flying off the craps table. _Oops!_ "Do over."

It's time to roll again. As I unconsciously chant my mantra, _Eight, eight, eight! C'mon, eight!_ I see a huddle of gamblers throw more money and chips on the table. I fling the dice. One hits a stack of chips and reveals a four; the other slowly hobbles along like a penguin. Before my mind can distinguish a number, I hear the Vegas stickman bark, "Seven ooooout!" My hopes—along with everyone's money—are swept away.

That's when my dad sat me down, at 21 years old, to teach me why people win and lose in craps—and in life.

Before I go on, you should know that my dad is lucky. Uncannily lucky. To him, slot machines are ATM machines. Once while waiting to collect his winnings on a slot machine, he casually put money in the machine next to it and won there, too. Now waiting to be paid on two machines (heck, what else is there to do?), he put money into a third machine. Yes . . . he won, again—three slot machines in a row all within a matter of minutes, each paying several thousand dollars! And that wasn't the first time, either. He also scored a $60,000 jackpot within minutes. *Badda bing, badda boom!*

But craps is his game. Countless times, I've seen players start with about the same amount of money, but before long, everyone is rationing their meager pile of chips while my father is stacking his piles high. What are his secrets to such extraordinary luck? *Nature is his role model.* After all, Nature has beaten the odds for more than four billion years.

Now before I share my dad's winning secrets, know that I'm using gambling here as a metaphor. Wherever the word *gambling* appears, you can substitute *career, love life,* or anything else in its place. Everything operates by the laws of Nature. As you'll see, training your mind and emotions to follow Mother Nature's winning example will create "luck" in your own life, allowing you to attract the results you want.

Nature's Law #1: Maintain Clear, Relaxed Focus

*"The observation of nature requires a certain purity of
mind that cannot be disturbed or pre-occupied by anything.
The beetle on the flower does not escape the child;
he has devoted all his senses to a single, simple interest;
and it never strikes him that, at the same moment, something
remarkable may be going on in the formation of the clouds
to distract his glances in that direction."*

— **Goethe**

My nervous, helter-skelter dice throwing, with a mind running amok and a mouth babbling unconsciously, meant one thing: I had no focus—and ultimately, no winnings.

"You must have a single-minded purpose. Simply focus on the game in the moment," my father advised. "Your goal should be to keep the dice together, hitting the middle back wall of the table. Just concentrate on getting the numbers to come up. And don't micromanage—be open to even better things happening!"

Dad was never obsessed about things taking place *exactly* his way. He was focused on the game, not the outcome. It's the only way to stay in the moment. After he stressed how important it was to be totally present, that notion became a game in itself. Before each roll, my cousin Cindy Wilkes and I would laughingly ask each other:

"Where are you?"

"Here!"

"What time is it?"

We'd shout in unison: "Now!"

Nature also teaches us to be present. Since a tiger can be lurking around any corner, a deer remains constantly alert. And as all predators search for prey, they maintain a razor-sharp focus. Unlike people, animals don't allow themselves to be constantly interrupted, nor do they multitask while on the hunt. They're completely present with a *single-mindedness of purpose.*

Nature's Secret Message
**Nature generally doesn't multitask;
she maintains a determined, sharp resolve.**

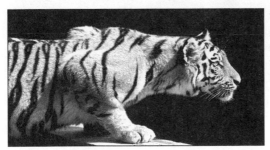

We could emulate the single-mindedness of the tiger, who stays in the present moment and does *not* multitask.

Humans, on the other hand, are masters of being unfocused. We multi-multitask (finding multiple ways to multitask). Rudolf Steiner believed that multitasking "blows one's circuits" and causes harm to the body's nerve-sense system—along with diminishing the joy and sense of peace in each action.

Best-selling author and leader in the field of mind-body medicine, Deepak Chopra, M.D., attributes quitting smoking to *not* multitasking. By being present with each puff on his cigarette and doing nothing else, he could begin to feel how his body didn't want it. His careful observation led him to gradually cut down, then eventually become a nonsmoker.

Studies show that simultaneously talking on the cell phone and driving causes an increase in automobile accidents. A different study, cited in the book *The 4-Hour Workweek,* showed that answering the phone and e-mails while also trying to get work done decreased a person's IQ by twice as much as smoking marijuana!

Still think multitasking is efficient?

One billionaire shared his secret with me for acquiring massive wealth: *laser-sharp focus.* I observed him in a meeting and was fascinated by his alert stillness. It was as if every pore in his body was open, listening and soaking up everything that enabled him to make a wise decision. Comparing it to the attentiveness of a hunting tiger, I call it "business stalking."

Legendary athlete Carl Lewis shares how his relaxed concentration helped him win nine Olympic gold medals:

> The calmest moments I ever had for a competition were just before I started, the last five seconds—when they would say, "Come to your mark." Instead of thinking about the race at that moment, that's when I would have the most intense meditation and focus. My mind would go blank, and my focus was just on the sound of the gun. There could be a million people there, someone could be screaming in my ear, and I wouldn't hear them. It would be so peaceful and calm. I went into, I guess, a deep form of meditation just before every competition because the last seconds were totally silent.[1]

Nature's Law #2: Allow and Trust

> *"Water gives life to the ten thousand things
> and does not strive."*
>
> — Tao Te Ching

After observing my tense, chaotic dice rolls, my dad remarked, "Relax. You're thinking too much and trying way too hard. It's almost impossible for money to get into a tightly closed fist. When you need it, you repel it. Instead, *allow* the money to come to you."

Coupling the first law (clear focus) with the second (allowing) combines feminine and masculine energies. The notion of allowing is deeply rooted in Nature: the sun rises and sets effortlessly, tides ebb and flow, grass grows, flowers unfold, and fruit ripens on trees—all in the natural rhythms of life.

Trusting in possibilities happens in Nature. Despite a cold winter, seeds still begin their journey upward through the soil, becoming seedlings that stretch toward the sky. Our fears and our calculations about all that could go wrong prevent us from trusting in the possibility of growth, change, and abundance.

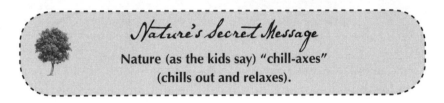

Nature's Secret Message

**Nature (as the kids say) "chill-axes"
(chills out and relaxes).**

I witnessed how these two laws of Nature can dramatically and instantly change the circumstances of a situation when I took a horse-training class. I mean *horse training,* literally, because in minutes the horse was training *me* to realize that even animals respond to clear energy that *allows* without struggle. The experience actually moved me to tears after I realized that the horse responded instantly to my inward state.

The idea was to lead the horse around the ring. However, the uninterested horse I was working with acted like he was stuck in glue. I couldn't get him to budge—even after numerous attempts to pull, pet, and coax him. The trainer-psychologist observed me closely and sized up the situation. He instructed me to stand back, breathe, and get clear on what I wanted to happen—and then *simply allow* the horse to go with me.

I stood back, took some slow, deep breaths, and made myself calm and still. Then I visualized myself confidently gliding the horse around the ring. Clarity washed over me. I picked up the rope and, with new confidence, started walking. It was as if someone had switched horses on me! Now the horse easily joined me, as if we were best friends. I wasn't trying, pleading, or pulling. The two of us were moving as one. It felt like a graceful dance as I led the gentle animal to walk, run, and gallop around the ring. I felt the power of clear intention and allowing—and doing so with effortless ease. The previously stubborn horse waltzed around the ring with a beautiful exchange of energy.

Here's another secret the horse taught me about winning and creating positive energy: after I visualized my goal (seeing and feeling the horse cooperating), I simply expected it to happen.

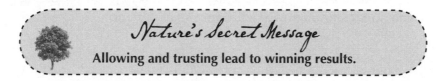

Nature's Secret Message
Allowing and trusting lead to winning results.

Some people don't expect to win in Vegas—or in life. I have a friend who tells everyone how lucky she is, and guess who always wins the raffles? She, like my dad, *expects* to win. The poem "My Wage," by the early-20th-century poet Jessie B. Rittenhouse sums up this point.

I bargained with Life for a penny,
And Life would pay no more,
However I begged at evening
When I counted my scanty store;
For Life is a just employer,
He gives you what you ask,
But once you have set the wages,
Why, you must bear the task.
I worked for a menial's hire,
Only to learn, dismayed,
That any wage I had asked of Life,
Life would have paid.

This poem is like the story of the man who dies and goes to heaven. He sees a room with everything you can imagine in it, then asks God why all those things aren't being used. God answers, "They were waiting to be given but the people didn't ask for, or expect them." British professor of psychology Richard Wiseman conducted a ten-year experiment on luck. He concluded that one of the principles of lucky people was a positive expectation.

Think of ways you can *allow* with *positive expectation.* For example, I watched my sister, a sleek athlete, lift weights with tensed hands and grimace as she loudly forced her breath between reps. Her trainer calmly whispered phrases like, "Relax your tongue. Relax your jaw. Relax your hands." Soon her movements and breath became as smooth and graceful as a ballet dancer. By releasing tension, letting go, she gained extra energy and power while also greatly improving her workouts.

During your workouts—or at any time of the day, no matter what you're doing—notice your tension, then gently breathe and relax into it. *Let go!*

Nature's Law #3: Face Your Fears

"Not everything that is faced can be changed;
but nothing can be changed until it is faced."

— James Baldwin

My dad would half-jokingly say about gambling, "The chips don't like scared energy. If you're afraid you'll lose your money— guess what will happen!" He added, "Most people are chanting something like *four, four, four,* believing it's positive thinking, but really it's dreadful hoping. They're fearful of getting a seven. If you're hoping to get an eight but afraid of getting a seven, what do you think you'll get? Fear overcomes hope. I've never seen a frightened winner." He finished by saying, "Once you let go of the fear, there's aliveness. Roll the dice, and know it's all gonna be all right."

Let's look at Nature: animals prey on fear. They can sense energy, whether it's fearful or calm. Many people have reported that they can venture unprotected into a swarm of bees and not get stung as long as they express love and don't generate fear.

Nature's Secret Message

Fear closes your heart. Be willing to let go of your fears and see what lessons Nature has for you when you make different choices.

Facing fears allows us to discover the lessons we need to learn and gives us access to a treasure of a wider perspective than we're able to achieve when we're gripped by this powerful emotion. Goethe, the German literary scholar, novelist, influential thinker, and scientist, used a creative approach to cure himself of an intense fear of heights. A cathedral in Strasbourg enthralled him. He studied it under different lighting conditions to sketch it, and he forced himself to climb the tower many times to help cure his phobia. It was as if he befriended the building through close study, intense observation, and experiencing it in as many ways as possible.

When he was about to leave the town, Goethe remarked to his friends that the tower was incomplete, and he went on to sketch how it would look when finished. It's fascinating to note that his drawing matched the original plans perfectly. People wondered who had given him this information, to which Goethe replied that the tower itself told him. He put so much attention and affection into observing it from every possible way that the tower's secret was revealed to him. Goethe befriended his fears and contemplated every aspect of them until finally he no longer felt afraid. He didn't ignore his fear; he dealt with it.

Goethe believed that if a person had a free, unbiased spirit of observation and sincere interest in something, then all of its mysteries would be revealed. Careful examination led him to access a deeper wisdom that went beyond the thinking mind in order to resolve his fears and make new discoveries.

Could we follow the ways of our ancestors who, like Goethe, took time to observe Nature's signs to find which plants, roots, or flowers to use as remedies? Or glean insight by watching how even inanimate objects can help solve our challenges?

Fear causes your mind to work on overdrive, obscuring your access to higher wisdom—right when you need it the most! By observing your fears, you become like the child who turns on the light to face the monster . . . and discovers that it's only a harmless robe hanging on a hook. So many times there's nothing real to fear.

Imagine yourself approaching your fears like Goethe did: with so much neutral observation, open-mindedness, and love that no room is left for fear. Could you roll up your sleeves, look right at a frightening (or uncomfortable) issue, find the blessings, and tap into your higher wisdom to address it? This positions you to gain a vast perspective and even deeper understanding. If you look at your emotional, physical, or health challenges in this manner, it would be much easier to figure out clear, wise solutions.

Meditation teacher Linda Lee, who trained at the Institut d'Orientation Psychologique in Paris for ten years and founded the nonprofit Pause Your Mind studio in Venice, California, offers a great approach for dealing with fear. She equates fear and worry to being in the slums of your mind and body. Why not travel to a higher place inside yourself? When consumed with fear, stop, breathe, and imagine yourself being elevated to a higher, lighter place inside. You can also ask for spiritual assistance to instantly raise your consciousness.[2]

Nature's Law #4: Be Happy and Playful

"Life's door, love's door, God's door—they all open when you are playful. They all become closed when you become serious."

— Osho

While watching people gamble, I've often wondered, *Are they happy because they're winning, or are they winning because they're happy?* On the other hand, what causes people to "seven-out" (lose) in Las Vegas? Let's start with a story to illustrate the lesson.

With an intense demeanor, a frantic woman pleads for help. She yells, "Shut up!" at her child so she can call someone to her rescue. Is this woman looking for an ambulance? No. She's at Home Depot, waiting for assistance in the paint aisle; however, her body registers her impatience and exasperation as a life-threatening emergency. Her tremendous stress generates a cascade of imbalance, starting with muscle tension and then moving into headache, poor digestion, and full-fledged anxiety. Her joy and energy evaporate, her mistakes compound, and her child starts to mirror her behavior.

If she were gambling, her negative energy would cause her to swiftly seven-out. Throughout many years of observing winners and losers in Vegas, I'm certain that anger, frustration, and negativity are *not* the traits of a winner. I've seen it far too often to be a coincidence. However, having fun and feeling genuinely happy energy *attracts* good fortune—in Vegas and in life. The expression "on a roll" says it all: winning creates positive energy, which helps us gain (or achieve) even more.

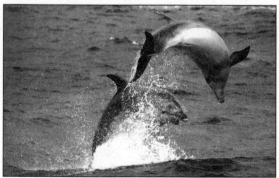

Animals play games and have fun!

Flowing energy, or what the Chinese call *chi,* is the essence of Nature. In her book *Beastly Behaviors,* Janine Benyus describes the playful behaviors of various animals, such as a dog fetching a ball or a dolphin playing a game of keep-away. (Dolphins even play a sexual game in which a male pushes objects around the tank with his penis.) Sea lions never tire of playing games, surfing, and leaping out of the water. Young gorillas spend most of the day playing and making chuckling noises. Pandas do somersaults! Beluga whales have a very playful nature as well. And squirrels chase each other, spiraling around trees, playing hide-and-seek or tag. They even make noises as if they're laughing.

You may think this free-spirited play is just for . . . play. Not so! Consider a recent episode of the television show *The Apprentice:* when one team member scolded the others for having fun, the mood of the entire group turned serious and tense. They began to brainstorm with their attention fixed on the deadline, rather than on their project. The show cut to the opposing team, whose members were enthusiastically and joyfully laughing and thinking up many ideas for their project. Both groups had the same deadline and task. Guess which team won? The free-spirited one! Throughout many episodes of this show, the teams that have the most fun and display the most cooperation repeatedly come out on top. The group that grows too serious, stressed out, and lost in conflict usually loses.

Clearly, finding the joy in work leads to better results. As Wolfgang Amadeus Mozart declared: "When I am, as it were, completely myself, entirely alone, and of good cheer; it is on such occasions that my ideas flow best and most abundantly."

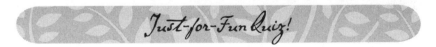

Just-for-Fun Quiz!

Test Your Nature IQ

Question: Do animals smile?

Answer: Yes! The mouth is the most expressive part of an animal's face.

Smiling

A Zen master by the name of Max Christensen tells us to put a smile on our face the whole time we meditate, so we don't take it so seriously. He explains that most people think of Zen masters as very solemn or stoic, but in reality, they place great importance on play and laughter. Christensen goes into long narratives about why this is vital and that people don't smile enough.

Did you know that smiling opens up the crown chakra at the top of your head? This is your direct energetic connection with the Divine. When you smile, you receive more benefits than you can imagine. This is another secret of Nature: smiling gives you power. A genuine outward smile will soon positively affect your internal state.

Nature's Secret Message
Wild animals play, enjoy life, and even smile.
We'd do well to emulate their playfulness.

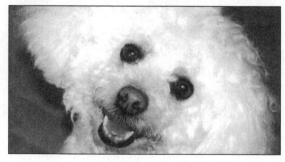

Animals' mouths can be very expressive.

Even animals smile! Desmond Morris, in his book *Animal Watching,* explains that animals' mouths are the most expressive part of their face. A slightly open mouth with lips pulled back, gently covering the teeth, is easily recognized as a smile.

Your smile keeps you healthy and happy, so treat yourself every day to something that makes you grin. While you're at it, laugh too, as that helps your digestive system. If you think of at least one thing that cracks you up each day, you'll give your internal organs a massage!

Christensen offers the analogy that if the village shaman gets sick, the entire village loses his wisdom. Therefore, before the shaman can help anyone else, he must first tend his own health and well-being. You may not be a shaman, but this is true for you, too.

"Winr-Winr-Winner!"

> *"When I am creating, the creating is the joy.*
> *The song coming, oh my God, what's this doing?*
> *It is writing itself. . . . All songs came like that;*
> *I was not trying. As soon as I tried, it went away."*

> **— John Lennon**

The looseness of play and not struggling, which is exhibited in Nature, is definitely a winning formula in Las Vegas. When I am fully present and enjoying myself, fear and worry take a temporary vacation and something amazing happens: I get lucky and win! I have more fun with a happy, playful mind-set, and even if I'm not always the winner . . . I still win because I'm having a great time.

After 84-year-old Josephine Crawford won ten million dollars on a nickel slot machine, she was asked if she felt lucky before she gambled that day. She replied, "I just love the *fun* of gambling. I go to have a fun time." Wise lady. Her tip also applies to winning in life!

As an ending note, if you're thinking about gambling, my dad also says that there are only two times when you should *not* gamble: 1. When you *need* the money. 2. When you *don't need* the money.

Applying Nature's Winning Principles

— *Bring yourself in the now.* Always start with the statement: *I am here.* Ground yourself and be present (especially if you feel nervous), look around the room, and start naming the colors and items you see, for example: "Orange rug, beige blinds, cream walls, bronze shelves . . ."

— *Observe Nature's effortlessness.* Repeat Linda Lee's mantra: *Today I do with less effort what I previously did with effort.* You can substitute the word *fear* in place of *effort,* or whatever it is you wish to change. Remember that love is fearless. Find the love in any situation.

— *Seek joy.* Ask yourself, *What nourishes my spirit?*

— *Find pleasure in doing.* Why not put a "to do" on your list that brings you pleasure? It can be something very simple, as long as it keeps those lighthearted juices flowing. Scientists are discovering that pleasure creates new neuropathways that can break old habits. Notice the relationship between feeling good and what's going on around you at the time.

— *Let go.* Do a body scan with your mind: relax your eyes, tongue, lips, jaw, shoulders, hands, abdomen, and legs . . . all the way down to your toes. Then go back to each body part and check to see if it's still relaxed. Discover where your "holding pattern" is, and breathe into that area to release the tension. Repeat this several times a day, and you'll notice a calmer, happier you.

— *Choose to relax.* This is vital, especially when you're under pressure or running late. By melting away tension and stress, you can deal with any pressing matter more effectively.

— *Have fun.* Always remember that enjoying yourself opens up your "clown" chakra.

❦ ❦ ❦   ❦ ❦ ❦

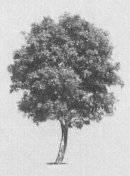

Part III

Nature's Secrets about
Our Spiritual Journey

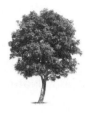

CHAPTER TEN

Nature's Patterns Aren't Random; Are Yours?

*"The universe appears to have been designed
by a pure mathematician."*

— **James Jeans**

The patterns we see in Nature offer us messages about our spiritual journey, on how we're intertwined with creation; and how to live richly, peacefully, and in balance. By observing the patterns in the natural world, we can begin to recognize the ones in our own lives, discovering the lessons we need to learn, our purpose, and our connections to others.

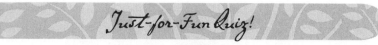

Just-for-Fun Quiz!

Test Your Nature IQ

1. Name four foods that naturally have star shapes in them or on them.

2. Can you identify where the tomato's star is?

3. Which common shapes are rare occurrences in Nature?

4. According to the Guinness World Records, what is the most number of times a person has been struck by lightning and survived?

5. Statistically speaking, which of the following is least likely to happen: getting struck by lightning, being in an airplane crash, or winning the lottery?

6. What one food never spoils and is made without any artificial preservatives or chemicals?

Answers

1. Blueberries, apples, star fruit, and tomatoes

2. On the stem, where it meets the tomato

3. A square and a right angle

4. Shenandoah National Park ranger Roy Sullivan survived seven lightning strikes (unfortunately, when he reportedly struck out in love, he killed himself).

5. Winning the lottery

6. Honey

Mother Nature Does the Math

- Are the shapes and patterns found in
  Nature coincidental?

- Do you think the numbers of leaves, petals, branches,
  and fruit are random, strewn about in a nonsensical
  order?

- Can mathematical principles be found in Nature?

- Do Nature's Shapes + Numbers = A Reflection
  of Divine Consciousness?

Mario Livio, an astrophysicist and author of the book *Is God A Mathematician?* points out that if you imagine a pin in the center of a six-sided snowflake, every time you rotate it by 60 degrees, you're going to get a snowflake that looks exactly the same. How the heck is a seemingly "simple" snowflake that perfectly constructed?

Michael Semprevivo invented PhiBar, a software program that applies phi relationships to the spectrum of colors, producing visually appealing combinations. He maintains: "God is in the numbers, or at least such a complex system did not and could not arise out of rocks banging together in space. My understanding of God is mathematical and geometrical in nature."[1]

Discussing math in Nature can take up volumes, and the conversation quickly becomes extremely complex. So I'll sum up a few basic concepts regarding numbers and shapes in Nature and the body.

Fibonacci, a number sequence that shows up in Nature with uncanny frequency, was developed as far back as 200 B.C., but Leonardo of Pisa (originally Leonardo Fibonacci) made it famous in the 1200s. The Fibonacci numbers are like Paris Hilton—they show up *everywhere*. This sequence can be found in music, science, the stock market, works of art, the human body . . . and *hidden in plain sight*, right in front of us in Nature. Here's the math:

If you're not a math aficionado, don't despair; I'll keep it simple. All you need to know about the Fibonacci sequence is that it's a specific order of these numbers: 0, 1, 1, 2, 3, 5, 8, 13, 21, 34, 55, 89, 144, 233, 377, 610, 987, and on it goes infinitely. (You can skip ahead to the paragraph after the numbers if you wish.) If you like math, here's how you calculate the Fibonacci numbers: start with 0 and add 1, then take the sum and add it to itself. Keep repeating and you get the Fibonacci number sequence. In other words, each new number is the sum of the two preceding numbers, as follows:

1 = 1 + 0
2 = 1 + 1
3 = 2 + 1
5 = 3 + 2
8 = 5 + 3
13 = 8 + 5
21 = 13 + 8
34 = 21 + 13
55 = 34 + 21

The Fibonacci sequence is used in the stock market, as Phil Riou, market analyst, writes:

> After the first few numbers in the sequence, the ratio of any number to the next number higher is approximately 0.618 to 1. . . . And the ratio of any number to the next lower number is approximately 1.618 to 1. (The higher one goes in the sequence, the closer the ratio becomes to this ideal ratio.) . . .
>
> The ratio between the Fibonacci sequence of numbers is known by the Latin name of *Phi*. It is also an irrational number with no ending: 0.618034. . . to infinity. *Phi* is also known as the Golden Ratio.[2]

How does this sequence of numbers relate to Nature? Flowers, leaves, and stems all contain Fibonacci sequences! It's fascinating to see that this really did "add up" as I counted some petals and leaves when I went outside to explore the concept. Now, for instance, it makes more sense to me why it can be hard to find a four-leaf clover. Four isn't a Fibonacci number. Of course, this isn't an exact rule of Nature; there are exceptions. However, the more you look, the more you'll find Fibonacci numbers.

Nature's Secret Message

The Creator must also be a mathematician, because life is made up of numbers appearing in splendid patterns.

Nature Paints by Number

Why do so many flowers have five petals, echoing the shape of a five-pointed star? Five is a Fibonacci number. Here's a small handful of the "stars" in Nature. Have you spotted this pattern before?

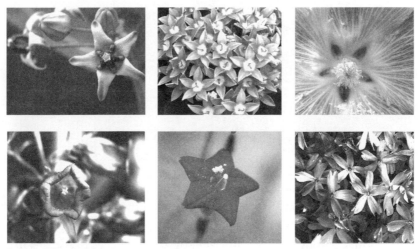

Seeing stars in Nature.

Examine the seed heads of plants that display the Fibonacci sequence, and you'll find that counting the leaves up and down the stem reveals the sequence. Look at the following illustration of the sneezewort plant, for example. The plant maintains the Fibonacci sequence at the "growing points," and the leaves also follow the pattern.

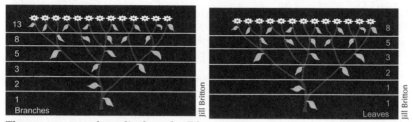

The sneezewort plant displays the Fibonacci sequence in its growth patterns.

Can you crack the pineapple's secret code? It looks rather ordinary, right? Look again, and think of the Fibonacci sequence. See what you come up with!

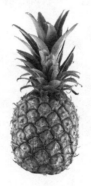

Jill Britton, a mathematics instructor at Camosun College in Victoria, British Columbia (who also created the illustrations of the sneezewort plant and pineapple), writes that pineapples have the Fibonacci code written all over them. Its hexagonal scales are also patterned into three distinct sets of spirals: one set of 5 spirals, a second set of 8 spirals, and the third set of 13 spirals, as show in the photos.[3]

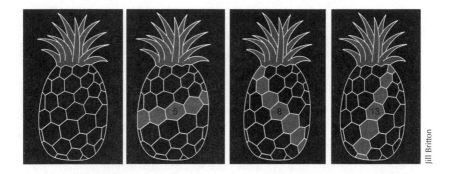

Think this is a coincidence? In a study conducted with 2,000 pineapples, not one deviated from the Fibonacci pattern.[4] But it gets even more interesting. Let's chart this numerical sequence on paper. And if you really don't like the math aspect, all you need to know is that the series creates a swirl. If you're curious, here's how the swirl was created.

Going back to the diagram of the sequence, it starts with one, which is one square high; then the sum is two, which is two squares high; then the sum of three, which is three squares high. Notice how the square's sides are successive Fibonacci numbers in length.

So what's the big deal about that? How does this relate to Nature? Well, if we draw a spiral, one quarter of a circle through each sum, we get something that looks like this:

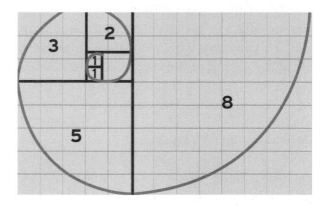

From this sequence, we get a spiral shape. Author and Phi expert Gary Meisner, "the Phi Guy," explains that Fibonacci numbers are related to spiral growth: "If you sum the squares of any series [pictured on previous page] of Fibonacci numbers, they will equal the last Fibonacci number used in the series times the next Fibonacci number. This property results in the Fibonacci spiral seen in everything from sea shells to galaxies."[5]

Phi (also known as the golden ratio), a number discovered in the fifth century B.C., is related to spirals as well. It begins with 1.6180339887. . . (and goes on forever). Some people feel that it represents "the reflection of Divine consciousness at work," "an outer ring of intelligence," or "the God presence in all living things." Author John Michael Greer says that the spiral "serves as a powerful image of the unfolding of what is hidden."[6] And Leslie Sloane, the color therapist and founder of Auracle's Colour Therapy, refers to phi as "the radiation of the heart," which may help explain why some people give roses to their loved ones on Valentine's Day. (Check out the swirl pattern of a rose in the upcoming photo.) And wouldn't you know, rose hips, the berrylike fruit of the rosebush, contain phytochemicals that protect against cardiovascular disease.

There are even references to it in the Bible. In Exodus 25:10, God commands Moses to build the Ark of the Covenant to hold his covenant with the Israelites (the Ten Commandments): "And they shall make an ark of acacia wood; two and a half cubits shall be its length, a cubit and a half its width, and a cubit and a half its height." Our "Phi Guy," Gary Meisner, provides insight into this verse: "The ratio of 2.5 to 1.5 is 1.666. . . which is as close to phi (1.618. . .) as you can come with such simple numbers and is certainly not visibly different to the eye."[5] Likewise, Gary also reveals that B-DNA (a form of DNA in the cell appearing as a double-stranded helix) and a DNA cross section are all based on phi.

If we examine the natural world, an astonishing 92 percent of plants displaying spirals or double whirls have Fibonacci patterns, according to Roger Jean, the author of *Phyllotaxis,* a book about the study of leaf arrangement.[7] (Jean surveyed 650 species in literature and 12,500 specimens in making this observation.) It's been said that Buddha once gave a teaching by simply holding out a rose, not speaking a single word. Is it a coincidence that the rose has this swirl, like phi? Was he teaching us to learn from Nature?

Before going any further, think of other swirl patterns you've seen in a natural setting. Even the rounded claws of numerous animals and the tusks of a walrus fit the phi proportions. How many can you name? Here are some examples:

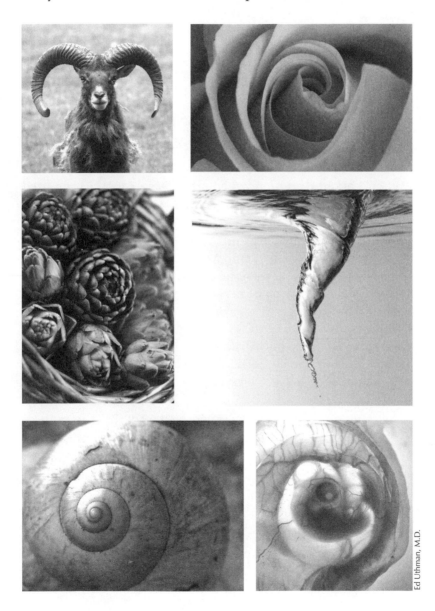

Ed Uthman, M.D.

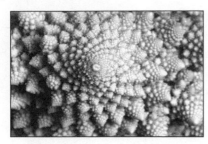
Notice the swirls on the cauliflower.

Nature's Art of Math

"Without mathematics there is no art."

— **Luca Pacioli**

When I asked world-renowned artist Dave Zaboski if he used phi in his art, he positively lit up, saying:

> I use it in everything I paint! I can't overstate its vital importance. The greatest artists throughout history have used the "Golden Mean." It's an energetic connection to all humans. Its effects are outside our ability to perceive, yet are harmonic to the human consciousness. We resonate with it. If you believe "what you see is what you get," then you're missing an entire universe of other energies and intelligences. It's beyond our subconscious mind, or as Jung calls it "the collective unconsciousness." Anyway you want to look at it—it's bigger than you are.[8]

This phenomenon even occurs in geometry. It's the ratio of the side of a pentagram to its diagonal. These diagonals cut into each other with the golden ratio, which yields a star shape. Market analyst Phil Riou points out that "joining the points of a pentagram (to make a pentagon) illustrates Fibonacci relationships between the lines. Also note that both these shapes are constructed around nature's most natural shape—a circle."[2] Have you ever thought about how the star has been such a powerful symbol throughout time and all over the world?

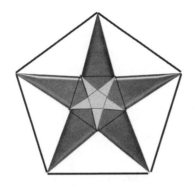

The mathematician Pythagoras called the five-pointed star the "symbol of his order." There are Fibonacci relationships occurring over and over.

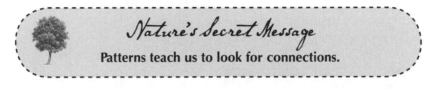

Nature's Secret Message

Patterns teach us to look for connections.

Seeing Stars—One of Nature's Favorite Shapes

I once listened to a radio show where a free-spirited woman said to the host, "There's a star in the apple." The host guffawed, and in a condescending tone, replied, "What?! I've never seen a *star* in an *apple!*" The woman demurely assured him that it was indeed there, but the host laughed at her claim. He'd eaten hundreds of *starless* apples.

That night, I was overtaken by curiosity and decided to look for myself. I walked into the kitchen and picked up an apple from the counter. I carefully observed it—inside and out—but didn't see the star. Was the host right?

Before you read any further, see if you can find the apple's star for yourself. Here's a hint: to uncover many of Nature's secrets, you need to see in new, uncommon, yet simple ways.

Ready for the answer? Slice an apple in half horizontally, between the top and bottom. Surprise! The star is in the core.

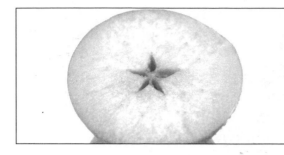

You get a star when you cut an apple in half horizontally.

Think of how many times you've cut an apple and completely missed the star, simply because you didn't think to cut it a different way. The apple's flower also contains a star. How many other "star-type wonders" could you be missing?

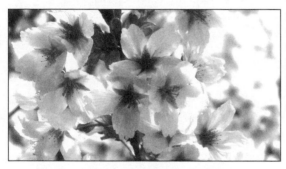

Folklore has it that if the flowers on fruit trees have stars, such as the apple flower [pictured], it means that the fruit is safe to eat.

Can you name other foods that have stars? There are a lot of them! You've probably looked at them hundreds of times but, like the radio host, didn't notice them.

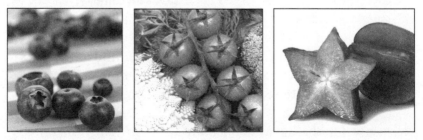

Nature's star-studded fruits.

How many times have you been out in Nature and noticed stars without looking at the sky?

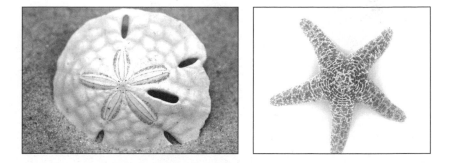

I used to wonder how people of ancient civilizations and early settlers knew what to eat (or not eat), as they lived entirely off the land. Was it all just trial and error? "Here, honey . . . go ahead, start dinner without me." Our ancestors would often observe which plants the animals did and didn't eat; and if they ate a particular plant, perhaps it was safe for human consumption, too. But they looked for other clues as well.

The ancients believed that a star on a fruit was an indication that it was safe for humans. The star was an important symbol because its five points represented our five senses. Did you know that generally many plants that have a five-petal flower and bear fruit are edible? In Chinese culture, the five elements (earth, metal, wood, fire, and air) are central to the balance of Nature, and they illustrate this as a *star*-shaped diagram. In his book *A Beginner's Guide to Constructing the Universe,* Michael Schneider describes the star throughout the ages as "the supreme symbol of life."

Do you notice anything else about the shape of a star? Each of the five parts replicates itself; they're all the same size. Now can you guess another way that the ancients related stars to the human body? Here's a clue: Take a look at the way in which the parts of a star and the human body line up in the following illustration:

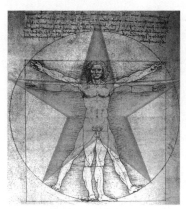

Ancient civilizations believed that the shape of the star was a powerful symbol in Nature, as well as representing the five senses of man.

Leonardo da Vinci's *Vitruvian Man* (pictured above) illustrates that the human body has mathematical proportions. Have you ever noticed that your palm is the width of your forehead? Your hand is also the length of your face. (Did you just put your hand up to your face to check and see? I bet they measure up!) And notice how your foot is about the same length as your forearm.

The five points of a star reminded our ancestors of the body in several other ways, too. Take a look at the illustration of the human body again and see how wondrously the phi sequence shows up:

- We have two arms, two legs, and a head.
- Our hands have four fingers and a thumb.
- Our feet have four small toes and a big toe.
- Our face has two eyes, two nostrils, and one mouth.

"How is it possible that mathematics, a product of human thought that is independent of experience, fits so excellently the objects of physical reality?"

— **Albert Einstein**

Nature's Wake-Up Call

Noticing Nature's symbols brings you more fully into the present and opens the door of awareness to receive deeper insights.

Think of how you unconsciously relate stars with wizards, magicians, celebrities, generals, mystics, mystery, success, and power. The star has some magic in it! It's also created on the order of phi proportions, the magic of which I discussed earlier. Stars hidden in plain sight could be Nature's way of saying, "Hey, wake up!" There are "awe-ha" moments all around you, if you become aware.

Think of how many times you quickly passed by a flower or sliced up an apple and missed its star. You may think, *So I didn't see any stars—no big deal. I'm too busy to notice such trivia! I have more important things on my mind.* But that's exactly the problem.

Have you heard the saying: "The time to relax is when you don't have time to relax?" When you're too busy, you can't really be fully in the moment. You're not able to see much. But by slowing down and becoming more present, you'll notice more clues around you and break the trance of busyness. Usually how you do one thing is an indication of how you do everything. If you're not paying attention in one area of your life, most likely you're not paying attention in other areas.

If you've missed so many of the stars around you (and in the form of your own body), what else are you overlooking? Is it possible that you're missing out on your surroundings, even people, because you're seeing everything in the same old way—preoccupied with thoughts about the past or future?

And speaking of not noticing, have you ever noticed the hexagon patterns around you?

The Hexagons Around Us

The hexagonal pattern appears in honeycombs and serves as the perfect holding container. Here's why: could *you* devise a way to store the most honey in the least amount of space? Bees did! And could *you* ensure that the honey wouldn't spoil, without the use of preservatives or chemicals? Bees did that, too.

Bees are "bee-yond" our comprehension. Philosopher Pliny the Elder said some ancients devoted their lives to unraveling the mystery of the bee. Humans would need to use elaborate calculations to determine that the waxy hexagonal pattern of the honeycomb was the ideal storage container.

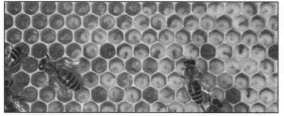

Every honeycomb is precisely constructed of hexagonal wax cells built by honeybees.

How do bees know to construct these precision-crafted structures? In his speech on patterns in art and Nature, science writer Philip Ball, Ph.D., summarizes: "They [bees] use another set of organs to engineer the thickness of the cell walls very accurately, to a tolerance of two-thousandths of a millimeter. They even manage to construct the correct tilt of the angle of the cell channel, which slants down at 13 degrees below the horizontal so that the honey doesn't run out."[9]

The hexagon is the most efficient shape they could use; circles would create gaps, which would waste space and wax, and could collect dirt. The hexagon shapes nest together perfectly with no gaps. Squares could be uncomfortable to use, and right angles are rarely found in Nature.

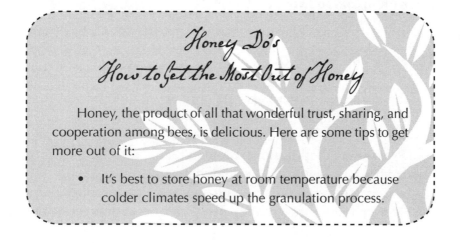

Honey Do's
How to Get the Most Out of Honey

Honey, the product of all that wonderful trust, sharing, and cooperation among bees, is delicious. Here are some tips to get more out of it:

- It's best to store honey at room temperature because colder climates speed up the granulation process.

- Granulation of honey is natural, so there's no need to throw it away if it crystallizes. You can reliquefy it by placing the jar in a warm-water bath until it returns to liquid form.

- Honey is a natural remedy for burns, rashes, and sore throats; and it can also be used as a facial mask.

- Natural honey is a healthy replacement for sugar, which is artificially processed.

Where else do we find hexagons in Nature? A water bubble has a hexagonal shape, as do many crystals, including rubies, sapphires, and emeralds.[10] The ice crystals of snowflakes are also arranged in a hexagonal pattern. "Snow water" has hexagonal structuring, and according to water expert, Mu Shik Jhon, Ph.D., it's highly energetic water that can slow the aging process, increase vitality, and prevent disease. Lowering the temperature of the water, he adds, helps to create a hexagonal structure.[11]

Hexagons are even found in space! In 1979, the *Voyager* was taking pictures of the mysterious planet Saturn. Scientists were astonished by an image of Saturn's north pole, revealing a perfectly shaped hexagon. In 2006, additional photos captured by the *Cassini-Huygens* craft confirmed the presence of this hexagon. Scientist Kevin Baines, Ph.D., of NASA's Jet Propulsion Laboratory, tells us that this pattern has existed for at least 20 years, and possibly much longer.

Just for fun, consider the similarity between popular images of extraterrestrials and the face of bees, with their large black eyes. Could the bees, with their extraordinary knowledge, be from "out of this world"? Yes, this may be a far-out (literally!) connection, but look at how they've devised things that we supposedly more intelligent beings are just now coming to understand.

Observing the myriad hexagons in Nature teaches us to become better observers in our own lives. If a hexagon can be very efficient, then we should ask ourselves: *Are we being efficient, or are we being wasteful—not valuing our resources, not being mindful, and not tending to what truly matters?* Recognizing the patterns in Nature teaches us to also recognize the patterns in our lives.

Another common pattern we often overlook is that of lightning, which has its own secret messages about the connection between earth and sky, as well as between our dreams for expansion and our need for roots.

"Lightning Up" . . . and Down: Patterns Above and Below

> *"Lightning is the root of the sky, transforming carbon and nitrogen into compounds assimilable for plants."*
>
> **— Robert Lawlor**

You may have seen Nature's spectacular fireworks—lightning—dozens of times, but have you ever looked beyond the brilliant flash of light to consider its mysterious, recurring patterns? This type of pattern, branching out in different directions, is a common design in Nature. Where else in the environment do you notice this design? Here's a hint: think "As above, so below."

Do the branching patterns of lightning remind you of plant roots? Let's spark your imagination and explore that similarity. The lightning pattern that echoes the appearance of roots illustrates how the sky and the earth are interconnected, just as you're interconnected with everything around you. That pattern is also shown in your veins, in trees, in embryos, and in rivers—many life-forms circulate in this pattern.

Both carry energy in many different directions. Robert Lawlor writes in his book *Sacred Geometry* that lightning and roots have similarities that are "functionally accurate." Like trees, lightning appears to have "branches" or "roots."

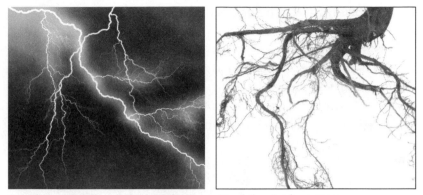

"As above, so below." Have you ever noticed the similar patterns of lightning [left] and a plant's roots?

Trees that are damaged by lightning usually have weak, shallow roots. The stronger and deeper the tree's roots are, the more energy it can disperse. Root systems ground a plant, allowing it to branch into the sky, growing and expanding. In order for your ideas to expand outward and flourish, they need roots, just as a plant does. And by the way, have you ever noticed how much of the upper part of a person's body is like the lower part? Obviously, the upper half has two arms with five fingers with the elbows in the middle, and the lower has two legs with five toes, with the knees in the middle. But if you look in an anatomy book, even the shape of the muscles in the upper and lower bodies mirror each other.

What other lessons can be learned from lightning, branches, and roots? It's intriguing to note that the powerful energy of a lightning storm releases water to the roots in the earth, and the plants in turn release the water back into the atmosphere. "In the Amazon forest," notes John Easterling, founder of the Amazon Herb Company, "50 percent of the moisture for rain is released directly from the trees. So, fewer trees means less rain."[12] Consider what you can learn from this aspect of Nature. Do you have a balance between giving and taking in your life? Are you living in harmony with yourself and others? All of these deeper, more spiritual questions arise when you start to pay closer attention to Nature's patterns.

"Brainstorming" on the Patterns in Lightning

Nature is a work of art, so let's examine the brushstrokes—the pattern of lightning. In addition to resembling roots, it also looks like the blood vessels of our bodies, the veins in our eyes, tree branches, the veins in leaves, and the meandering shape of a river. Notice how all of these patterns have life moving through them.

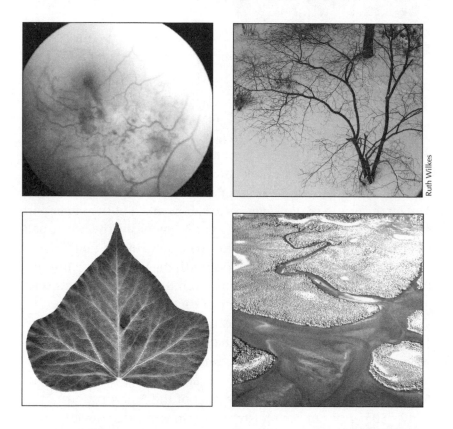

Ruth Wilkes

Like lightning, these patterns disperse the energy of life: roots move vitamins and nutrients from the earth into the plant; the body's veins move nutrients to the cells; branches and leaves move energy to and from the trees; and rivers move flowing water from their source ultimately to the ocean. Are these similarities just coincidence? Could these patterns represent something or be some sort of secret code, informing us about movement and sharing? If blood and oxygen cease to move through our bodies, we die. What conclusions can we draw about trying to hold on to what we have, never expanding, moving, or sharing?

Roots teach us to look at what lies hidden beneath our thoughts and actions and at what's supporting us. Are we drawing upon wisdom and strength, using deep roots? Or are we barely supporting ourselves? Roots that push through obstacles serve as a metaphor for what we can do if we take our time and focus on how we want to grow.

Do *your* roots run deep? Do your spiritual or health practices help you reach higher?

Notice how roots "branch out." As in life, things don't move in a straight line, and at times they can throw you a sharp curve. Could you flow like the curves of these patterns, which may be a more natural approach to life, rather than the "straight line" approach?

"Square Roots"—Not Common Patterns in Nature

"Nature's messages are like poetry," says herbalist and author Matthew Wood. They can be complex, subtle, and interwoven. Just like a person, many aspects exist for us to observe and understand.

Think of how few square shapes you see in a natural setting. Wood reveals that Nature abhors a square shape or 90 degree angle—which is actually quite unnatural. In herbology, these shapes are considered separate from Nature. He states: "You don't see 90 degree angles in the plant kingdom very often. But every once in a while you do; then it's usually a signature for someone with a strong personality totally dominated by ego—a person alienated or separate from nature."[13]

Wood points to a plant called the werewolf root (*Apocynum androsaemifolium*), also called "spreading dogbane" or north and south root, as the plant spreads at 90 degree angles both above and below ground. And wouldn't you know that it's used as a remedy to help people make tough decisions. This is extremely powerful—so do *not* try this at home! It requires the supervision of an experienced herbalist, as the herb can also play tricks with your mind.

So you can learn by observing not only what you and other people do, but also what the roots do. I've seen some roots so strong that people used them as stepping-stones and others strong enough to actually crack cement.

Roots are only one way to discover Nature's secrets in trees. You can also get more clues from observing other parts of the tree. For more insights, remember that what a plant does in Nature, it may also do in your body.

How Something Functions in Nature Reflects How It Can Function in the Body

Earlier, we looked at walnuts and their similarities to the brain, but the walnut tree itself holds secret messages, too—ones that help us make sense of our lives. Nature's signs often fit together like puzzles. We can carefully look at all the parts to see how the pieces fit. We can even check studies or go by our intuition to confirm what we've observed, and watch as everything falls into place.

> *Nature's Secret Message*
>
> **Observe what a plant does and how it interacts with the rest of Nature. Then ask yourself,**
> *What lesson about behavior and interaction does this plant offer?*

"Walnut trees are attacked by some 64 diseases and 296 species of insects and mites," asserts garden expert Tom Clothier. Yet these trees are very hardy. Professor Emeritus Walter Beineke, Ph.D., explains that both the husk's thickness and its juglone (a toxic compound occurring naturally in black walnut trees) prevent parasites from getting at the walnut meat. If juglone protects the tree from parasites, could it also kill parasites in humans? Yes! Black walnut is a common and popular parasite remedy used in many modern formulas. More than that, walnut trees tell us that living in harmony with Nature means that we must also have ways to guard against that which might drain or harm us. Walnut trees are sturdy and strong, and the casings for their seeds are thick, protecting what is of value—its life and ability to procreate.

We looked at how Nature relates to us. Now let's look at her symbolism.

Nature's Signs Are Everywhere

The more we pay attention to Nature, the more attuned we'll be to her signs. We'll start noticing and thinking about the connections in our own lives. Symbols can be quite powerful communicators, speaking straight to our right, intuitive brain. We use them in everything from advertising to religion, and they even show up in our dreams. They have both universal and personal meanings.

In her book *Learn to See*, Mary Jo McCabe explains how one's higher self, or inner guidance, speaks in symbols that we can recognize if we open ourselves to this universal library of knowledge. She asks, "Why live in two dimensions only? If you identify yourself only by what your conscious self tells you, you miss the power open to you and live a condensation of life." Carl Jung also wrote a great deal about symbolism. In *Man and His Symbols,* he states: "There are numerous well-authenticated stories of clocks stopping at the moment of their owner's death; one was the pendulum clock in the palace of Frederick the Great at Sans Souci, which stopped when the emperor died."

I experienced this type of symbolism firsthand. When my dad was in a Wisconsin hospital undergoing angioplasty, I was in Los Angeles, working at my computer. Suddenly, all the power in my building went out. At that moment, it was like time stopped—it was eerily still. I instantly knew something was wrong with my dad. I knelt down and prayed for him to live. The power in the building seemed to be struggling to restore itself, mirroring what I sensed with my dad. I frantically thought, *C'mon, c'mon!*

Finally in one gush, the power came on—and I knew my dad was okay. I put my head down and kept saying, "Thank you, thank you, thank you." All of this happened without any thought on my part—just an intuitive knowing that something was wrong.

When I finally got a call through to the hospital, I discovered that the surgeon had accidentally severed three arteries while pulling the catheter out, forcing my dad into an emergency triple bypass. My father later reported floating above his body, counting the people who hurriedly wheeled him into heart surgery. Later when I went to reset the clocks that had stopped during the power failure, I noticed that they'd stopped at the same time my dad was rushed into emergency surgery.

My mom also once remarked to me that the vacuum cleaner her sister had given her had stopped working on the day my aunt died. Another coincidence?

At a lecture I'd attended, author and shamanic practitioner Steven Farmer, Ph.D., told of the day he was sitting at his desk, wondering if he should do a singing project, when suddenly a huge grasshopper leaped onto his computer. He took that as a sign to "leap in" and do the project, especially since he knew that grasshoppers are known for singing.

Nature's Secret Message
Just like Nature, our lives contain many hidden symbols and patterns that, if we discover and examine them, can help us grow and flourish. Recognizing this is vital to positive change.

What if you aren't noticing any signs or patterns? Here's an exercise to help you become fully present so that you can spot the symbols, clues, and synchronicities in your life: Think of a question that you really want answered. For this exercise, it's best to pick only one question. Pay attention over the coming days, and watch for clues to your answer. These don't have to be clues you'll find in Nature. They may be clues in your environment (on the street, in your home, in your car, and so on), or they could be auditory clues (a snippet of a song that answers your question or a word you overhear as you're tuning your radio to find a station).

Here's an example from my own experience. Once I was trying to decide if a certain project would be beneficial for me. The answer was very important to me so I asked for a sign to show me if I should go ahead with it. A short time later as I was walking home, a beautiful three-inch canary yellow butterfly whooshed by, almost touching my nose. I gasped at its unusual beauty! Instantly, a good feeling swept over me, and I felt that it was a positive sign of change . . . but later on, doubts started to creep in. *It was just a coincidence,* I told myself, even though I hadn't seen a butterfly like that in my entire life. *No, I really need some guidance, a sure sign to help me with this important decision.*

The following morning, I was walking through the parking lot of a huge shopping mall. The bright sun reflected off a shiny object on the pavement, just in front of my car door. It was so bright that it was like a mirror in the sun. I picked it up—a beautiful medallion with a raised image of a basket of fruit, inscribed with the words *Expect Miracles.* The project I was deciding about dealt with food, too.

When I saw it, a knowing came over me. *Yes, it was the right project.*

How do you know what's really a clue for you? Stay aware of the combination of your outer surroundings and inner feelings. You'll find many answers where these two areas intersect. You may feel an inner knowing or a "pull" in your gut or heart. Often it's simply a sense that something is or isn't for you. Notice how your body responds when you think of the issue. If you tense up, it may not be for you. If you feel spaciousness in your body and breathe easily, that can be a positive sign to go for it.

The more you pay attention to yourself and your surroundings, the more insights you'll gain. Like the stars, these signs are small ways to get in touch with your inner knowing and feelings. Take time to observe your environment and recognize subtle clues in the ways that the ancients did. Go ahead—see what magical discoveries are in the stars for *you.*

"Never give up on your dreams—follow the signs."

— **Paulo Coelho**

Here are some highlights to remember about Nature's math and patterns from permaculturist Jeanette Aguilar:

- These patterns connect us to Mother Nature.

- This awareness of sacred geometry takes the human spirit to a higher vibration level, attracting other people with a higher level of integrity.

- When we become aware of the intrinsic patterns in our lives, we come to a realization that all life is sacred. We become connected to all things in the universe.[14]

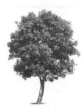

CHAPTER ELEVEN

----

*Communicating with
Nature, Up Close and Personal*

*"I love to think of nature as an unlimited
broadcasting system through which God speaks
to us every hour, if we will only tune in."*

— **George Washington Carver**

How do you think medicine men, indigenous healers, and shamans came up with powerful remedies when they didn't have studies and research findings, media news flashes, pharmaceuticals, or medical texts to consult? They believed that they communicated with the plant spirits, receiving guidance as to which plants or herbs would heal a person.

These wise sages retreated into Nature because they trusted that the earth reveals everything. One thing that the ancient healers had in common was their reverence for all living beings; they understood that plants have much to offer us about healing on all levels of reality: physical, mental, emotional, and spiritual. Do we subconsciously pick up on this, too?

Our Love Affair with Plants

Our love of Nature is visible all around us—in plain sight. Nurseries are brimming with a wide variety of plants and colorful flowers just waiting to grace our homes; and millions of people around the globe find gardening remarkably pleasurable, rewarding, and even spiritual. A popular garden ornament is a stone carved with the words: "God is nearer to us in a garden than anywhere else on Earth."

Getting our hands in the earth and connecting with it can have profound effects on the mind and body. Many accounts detail how gardening helps depressed people, and studies even show that it also has a calming effect on violent prisoners. It's not surprising! (Remember that in Chapter 6, we talked about the ways in which the ground, grass, and dirt—as well as the ocean and sand—can dissipate negative energies.)

When we enter a grocery store, we're usually greeted by a large assortment of irresistible, colorful bouquets. Flower shops throughout the world abound with floral arrangements for every occasion, as almost all of our ceremonies include flowers, such as at times of birth, marriage, death, initiations, and romance. Oh, the magic of flowers!

Let's dig a little deeper. Could it be possible that we have a greater connection to plants? Do they do more than put us in a good mood because they're pretty? Are we so deeply interconnected with plants that we can feel their energy even as they feel ours? If this were true, what would it say about our relationship to all of creation, and to all of the world's creatures?

We all know people who seem to have a green thumb. My grandmother, who came from a farming background in Europe, brought her love of Nature to America. She became the "plant doctor" in the neighborhood, with women bringing her their sick and dying plants so she could restore them to health. When friends would comment on her skills, she'd laugh, saying, "No, I just love to take care of plants." Was it the love in her healing touch that plants responded to? Was she in tune with what her "patients" needed, intuiting how much water and sun they required? We know that plants bend toward the sun for energy, but what other aspects of their environment do they respond to? How do we influence them, and how do they influence us?

Plant Communication

Janine M. Benyus, the author of *Biomimicry,* describes how Nature far exceeds some of mankind's best ideas:

> Our inventions have already appeared in nature in a more elegant form and at a lot less cost to the planet. Our most clever architectural struts and beams are already featured in lily pads and bamboo stems. Our central heating and air-conditioning are bested by the termite tower's steady 86 degrees F. Our most stealthy radar is hard of hearing compared to the bat's multifrequency transmission. And our new "smart materials" can't hold a candle to the dolphin's skin or butterfly's proboscis.[1]

Nature comes fully loaded with brilliant creations that are more complex than we can imagine. Plants can appear simply beautiful, but they're actually chemically complex. In fact, studies show that they have "intelligence." Anthony Trewavas, a professor at the University of Edinburgh and fellow of the Royal Society of Edinburgh, reports that plants detect light, water, temperature, chemicals, vibrations, gravity, and sounds. "A plant knows to release perfumed scents to attract pollinators, yet can send out toxic smells to repel insects and predators," he explains. "Plants can also create chemicals to heal and protect themselves when harmed. In some plants, one damaged leaf sets off a chemical chain reaction that helps protect the rest of the leaves."[2]

The following photos by professor and researcher Eshel Ben-Jacob show the colony structures that bacteria form as adaptive responses to laboratory-imposed stresses designed to mimic hostile environments that occur in Nature. The structures are, quite literally, works of art that have been exhibited in museums.

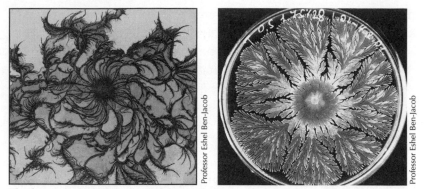

The bacteria pattern's organization illustrates the social intelligence of bacteria and how they are cooperative organisms leading complex social lives.

Unlike animals or weather, plants often don't get our attention because they're not nudging us. We see an animal moving and instantly get excited, but plants can become like wallpaper, ignored even when they're resplendent in their beauty. We perceive that we're too busy to be spending time getting to know plants and can't imagine how they can interact with us. However, slowing down and observing Nature will allow us to recognize just how much plants have to "say" to us.

Years ago, I kept hearing that people communicate with plants. It sounded far-fetched, and I'd joke with my friends, "They're fluent in many languages—oak, pine, birch . . ." but then I discovered that the cytogeneticist and Nobel laureate Barbara McClintock *asked* plants to solve specific problems for her. And George Washington Carver, who made the peanut famous, said it was the peanut itself that gave him advice on all its uses. Native American scholar Timothy Jenks, Ph.D., told me that medicine men would contact the plant's spirit for advice on which remedy to choose. Some aborigines also speak with plants' spirits. *Huh?* I wondered. *Is it really possible to communicate with Nature?*

The revelation that a plant is a living, communicating being was planted in my mind years ago, at my friend Joe's deathbed. He was vibrant, charismatic, and head-turning handsome. He had survived living with AIDS for ten years—nine years longer than his doctor's prognosis. A very spiritual man, Joe felt that drugs would hinder his soul's progress. Therefore, although he experienced excruciating pain, he didn't even take aspirin.

I was with him on his birthday, which also happened to be the last day of his life. His body resembled a brittle tree in winter, stripped of color and leaves, but alive with a deep, quiet sense of peace. His hospice room was filled with birthday gifts of lively plants. Joe could hardly speak, but words weren't needed. Our silence was intimate.

A caretaker came in to announce the end of visiting hours. I quickly reminded Joe how much he was loved, referring to all the plants that filled his tiny room. He murmured, "It's so beautiful how they communicate, isn't it?"

Confused, I blurted out, "Wha—what do you mean?" He managed to get out the words: "I love how they dance." He then barely whispered, "They're . . . *so* loving."

As I walked out into the chilly night, my friend's words swirled in my mind. Was he hallucinating, even though he wasn't on drugs? Does the mind play tricks to help ease the pain? Or could Joe have seen something—another dimension? I didn't know, but I was comforted by the fact that he felt a loving presence in his solitary room, whether real or imagined.

This experience opened my mind. I had no idea how passionate some people were about plants and how deep their belief was that we could communicate with them until I began to hear numerous stories of people communing with Nature. For example, Timothy Jenks, Ph.D., recounts:

> I went to visit my friend Peter, a shaman who lives in the country. To teach me a lesson in listening, he took me to a huge hickory tree in the woods and told me to tune out other distractions, and open myself to a vibration or sense that flows between a plant and me.
>
> It took some time to quiet my mind and focus on the tree, and then to just wait. Eventually, I heard—or perhaps sensed— a whispered, "Welcome to my family," and looked up at the esnormous trunk and branches. I noticed that branches crossed and intertwined with branches from other trees, also hickories,

and suddenly realized that the family of trees extended for acres. I did not hear him speak with my ears, but I *felt* him standing for centuries in that place, and I felt love and connection for the other trees and to me.[3]

Can we commune with Nature, sense our energy connection with it, and draw from its strength and wisdom by intuiting its guidance?

Going Out on a Limb

Are we all part of a vast field of consciousness, which could allow communication with Nature? Cultures throughout the world and all through time have communicated with plants; in fact, shamans, medicine men, and indigenous healers would journey inside the plant and respectfully commune with its spirit. Native Americans conducted ceremonies and used their dreams to get in touch with the plant kingdom. Many ancient cultures believed that fruit was love showered upon them as gifts from God. In order to give back, they'd take the seeds from the fruit and return them to the ground to continue the cycle. Native Americans would place tobacco or a hair from their head on the ground as a harmonious offering before uprooting plants to build on the land. Ripping out the trees and plants without first making an offering would have been seen as terribly disrespectful.

Herbalists often speak to plants to explain the purpose for picking them, believing that the plants connect with the vibration of energy coming from their gesture. Other cultures will purposely leave the fruit on certain trees as a show of respect, and to show that they aren't taking everything. This can be seen as similar to tithing.

Nature researcher, author, and teacher Machaelle Wright attributes the success of Perelandra, her world-renown nature research center in Virginia, to speaking with the plant spirits. She even uses applied kinesiology (tests on the electrical network of a living system, also called "muscle testing") on her garden to decide which nutrients (and how much of each) to add to each plant. She proposes the idea that we team up with Nature's intelligence to produce an equal partnership that will enrich our lives and that of the planet.

I began to discover even more stories of everyday people connecting with Nature. At first I thought these folks might need to speak with a therapist instead of a plant, but after hearing so many independent stories with familiar threads, I began to think, *Do all of these people have active imaginations, or could they actually be communing with Nature?* I noticed that, generally, those who claimed that they connected with Nature felt better for doing so and were able to "get out of their own way."

I interviewed Amita Welles, an intuitive who has worked with the Lakota Deer Tribe and other indigenous people, and she describes communing with Nature as opening up and really listening with gratitude and humility to all of the life around us. She believes that when we get ourselves out of the way (becoming still and emptying our minds), we create an inner peacefullness that enables us to see, feel, and sense in more profound ways, and to even hear what plants can communicate. When we stop trying and simply allow is when we create those "Aha!" moments, which occur when we really see what has always been right in front of our eyes. This happens as we reopen our hearts and hear our inner voice with love and compassion. Shifting within allows safe passage for other discoveries and reconnections within our being with Nature and with all life in general.

Amita emphasizes that emotional garbage or intense feelings can sometimes get in the way and prevent us from fully being given or receiving the help we need from the plants, or the stewards of the earth, as she calls them. They're the wisdom keepers because they've learned how to survive and thrive in their environment, and they carry this knowledge within them.

We're all carrying this wisdom within each of us as well. We've just forgotten our connection to the earth and our place within her. Collectively, we're in a time of deep reawakening and reassessing our "magnificence" as an all-powerful species on our planet as we experience the effects of our actions upon all life. Communicating with plants and Nature requires patience, for we're undoing what we've been taught, which is *to do* versus *to be* and to ignore our inner voice.

When we listen to our own quiet voice, we begin to hear the other voices of life communing with us. Love simply is. There's enough in the world to fill all of us amply, if we so desire. Once we stop allowing the ego to make our choices, we see and experience the world around us in a more conscious, divine way. It becomes a mirror reflecting our true nature back to us, illuminating our power through our intentions, thoughts, feelings, words, and actions in creating our reality and life experiences. This flow of shifting and aligning continues to expand and transform as we open our heart of hearts and accept the oneness of all life.[4]

Permaculturist Jeanette Aguilar beautifully expresses her experience of oneness with Nature:

> I was watering a patch of blueberries, when a hummingbird flew next to my hand. I stood very still so it would not be frightened of my presence. It let me know that it needed to take a shower. I moved the hose away from the fence so it could get to the water flowing. It flew about three inches from my hand and took a two or three minute shower. I could have petted it if I wanted to. It wasn't even afraid to be that close to me. It had so many beautiful colors, reminiscent of a brilliant fire opal and iridescent greens and browns. By the time it was done showering, it rested itself on the fence about 12 inches away from me, shook itself dry, rubbed itself against the fence, and rested for a little bit. Then it flew away like lightning.
>
> It was such an amazing experience to be that close to one of God's beautiful creatures. I felt so blessed by the moment; I had to share the blessing with you.[5]

Nature's Secret Message

We may not always be able to see Nature's flow of energy, but we can sense it if we pay close attention, and we can learn what it has to teach us.

Former professor and Taoist master Robert Kuang Ju Wu explains that traditional Taoist masters often live in mountains and wooded areas in order to be one with and energized by Nature. They won't live in cities since this disconnection from the natural world may cause them to become detached from their wisdom. Kuang Ju adds that anyone can feel energized in Nature simply by standing in front of a tree, assuming a particular Qigong position, and breathing in a certain way. Zen master Max Christensen further asserts that the Taoist way is to immerse yourself directly in Nature—allowing a merging with the trees, land, and sky—because Nature has the answers. The more you tune in, the more you're reminded that you're an energy being, intricately connected to the earth.

"Can You Hear Me Now?"

> *"Learning is experience.*
> *Everything else is information."*
>
> — **Albert Einstein**

Since everyone differs in how they learn and find answers, I've included the following exercises for gaining clarity and connecting with Nature's wisdom. Wilderness guide and author Steven Harper adds that communing with Nature may take time and understanding, and honing a relationship with the earth is just like building a relationship with a person.

When you learn to listen to Mother Nature's subtle messages and pick up on her energy, you'll soon realize that you've learned to listen to people better, too. You'll recognize what they're communicating nonverbally, and you'll discover that by tuning in to what's happening around you, you can access far more wisdom than if you merely tried to analyze and think through what to do and how to interact with others.

"Plant's Search for Meaning"
by Joanne Cohen, a certified herbalist who has a private
practice that's rooted in botanical medicine

Appreciating a plant is very similar to forging a relationship with a person. Just like people, every plant has a personality with unique qualities. The only way we create deeper relationships in our day-to-day lives is to spend time with others.

Pick a plant you feel drawn to, and look at its surroundings. Get to know where it lives. What's the soil like, how much sun does it receive, what color are its flower (if it has any), what bugs are attracted to it, and what other plants are growing nearby? All of these qualities lend to understanding the plant, to discovering its remedies, and even possibly comprehending more about yourself.

By merely sitting with a plant and feeling a deep appreciation for the presence of all plants on this Earth, you'll notice details that you may not have ever noticed. People have reported hearing sounds, words, or messages; seeing images around the plant; or receiving an intuitive feeling about its essence.[6]

Sensing Energy

Does your food emit an energy that you can feel? Hold some food in your hand, tune in to your body, and see if you can sense or feel anything. I've heard people say that they can actually feel the difference between organic and nonorganic foods. They also choose this exercise to intuit if the food is beneficial for them.

You can use this exercise to sense the energy of other people as well. Shut down your thoughts for a minute, and tune in to another person. What impressions can you pick up about that person? It's amazing how much information you can receive by observing and tapping into your senses.

Using Nature Imagery to Gain Clarity
by intuitive Karen Seeberg, the founder of The
Energy Centre in Pacific Palisades, California

When faced with a decision, try this exercise to help you gain clarity by drawing upon Nature's wisdom:

1. Breathe deeply. Close your eyes, and inhale and exhale three to five times.

2. Use your imagination to picture any blank screen: computer monitor, TV, movie screen, or empty stage.

3. Focus on your situation of concern—any health challenge, job issue, relationship question, money matter, or other topic that requires action or a decision.

4. Now visualize this issue on your "screen" as something that grows in Nature, such as a tree, bush, or flower. Once an image begins to form, take a few moments to watch the screen for more details to fill in. For example, if you visualize the issue as a tree, look around for the sky, ground, and surrounding foliage. Pay close attention to the details and any symbolic meaning they may have, and ask yourself more in-depth questions, such as:

   - Does my tree have a large, sturdy trunk (a solid position)?

   - Do the roots run deep and wide (potential financial abundance)?

   - Are there birds nesting in the branches (can it feed and nurture others)?

   - Is the sun shining on it (does it have higher guidance, integrity)?

   - Are the leaves vibrant or pocked where aphids have nibbled at them (indicating a vital or deficient company)?

- Is the sky dark and overcast or crystal clear?

- Is the landscape inviting?

5. Finally, imagine the wind blowing across this scene, and note your surroundings.

   - What happens to the leaves? Do they sway (showing flexibility and resilience)? Do they fall off (revealing weakness)?

As you interpret the details, you'll develop a sense of what you need to do. A full, lush garden; dried-up leaves and frail branches; or an influx of nonnative species are metaphors that convey deeper meanings for you. The language of Nature transcends the intellect and speaks directly to your heart.[7]

I did this exercise with a friend who couldn't decide if a new job was right for her. She took a minute to relax and picture a blank screen in her mind. Then I said, "Think of this job and describe the first Nature scene that pops up in your mind." She quickly replied, "Oh, I see a scene from Africa! It's sunny out, and lions are lying around below a low tree." She explained this exotic scene a bit further, and then I said, "Now walk into the scene to see how it feels." These words abruptly slipped out of her mouth: "Oh God no—there are lions there!"

It took a second for us to realize her unconscious statement, and then we burst out laughing. A knowing suddenly came over her that the job wasn't right, realizing all the demanding work at this lovely place may eat her alive.

Walking in Nature for Answers

You may find the answers you seek to challenges in your life by experiencing how the Native American Indian connects to Nature. Susan Teton, the author of *Medicine Teachings*, demonstrates how the four directions—north, south, east, and west—used in a "medicine walk" cover the physical, emotional, mental, and spiritual aspects of an issue; along with the four seasons, the four stages of life, and the four times of the day (dawn, noon, evening, and night). The Native American traditional "medicine" uses sacred symbolism found in the uniqueness of everything in Nature.

To begin, pick a place that feels inviting. Create a sacred space with a circle that shows the four directions. Begin in the center of the circle with a clear intention, and ask Nature to help you find solutions. When you're ready, walk to the east.

— **East** is the direction of the rising sun, sending energy toward a new or existing endeavor. It represents your spiritual side and the playfulness of a child. Allow Nature to communicate with the lively child in you. Use your intuition and wait to see what captures your attention. Is there anything symbolic that calls to you? Once you receive the medicine (or insight), express gratitude and walk to the next direction, the south.

— **South** represents the heat of midday and signifies passion, sex, courage, and emotions. What insights are you aware of? Give thanks for this encounter and walk to the west.

— **West** is the place for contemplation and reflection. When daylight fades, it's time to rest so that you can replenish. It represents your physical side. Listen for new insights from Nature. Receive her gift with thanks and walk to the north.

— **North** is the home of winter and the elder, each with a crown of white, symbolized by wisdom, healing, and your mental side. Breathe in the healing power of faith and listen. Receive new strengths and go back to the east to close your circle. Then return to the center to complete your walk and give gratitude for the "medicine" received.[8]

Record your experience in a journal and remain open. You may also receive insights later in various ways, including in your dreams. Nature gives us "medicine" so we can go deeper into healing an issue. She also has a lot to teach us about how to deal with change.

People from every culture have explored ways to connect to Nature. Whether these efforts resonate with you or not, they're all marked by a profound respect for the forces of Mother Nature. And it's possible that plants respond to respect and love, just like animals and people do. Let's now look at what we can learn from Nature regarding change.

Nature's Messages on Change

We often fear and resist change, but we need to learn from Nature's ability to constantly regenerate and renew. The resilient weeping willow and the rhythmic ebb and flow of tides teach us about being flexible and successfully adapting to change.

It reminds me of the saying, "Nothing is carved in stone," for Nature is always changing. A seed becomes a plant, a bud opens to form a perfect flower, and each season charms us with its own colors and weather patterns.

How do you deal with change?
How does Nature deal with change?
Any difference?

How do you feel when change suddenly arrives at your doorstep without an invitation? Does it seem like an unnatural occurrence? Have you spent a lot of time and energy desperately running, avoiding, and resisting change . . . only to eventually realize that it was for the best?

Close friends once unexpectedly showed up at my house for Christmas dinner. Their flight had been canceled that morning, which had upset all of their holiday plans. Throughout the meal, I noticed that my friend was agitated. She couldn't savor the delicious food or enter into the holiday spirit. Her husband, on the other hand, was jovial and relaxed, thoroughly enjoying the moment.

At the end of the evening, she finally blurted out, "I just don't do well with change!" to which everyone seemed to nod with great compassion, as if saying, "Who does?"

Her response reminded me of my friend Paul, a high-powered businessman who flew the New York–Los Angeles route several times a month. On one occasion, his usually prompt driver was caught in heavy traffic, causing Paul to miss his flight by only a few minutes. He was livid. Back at home, he continued to feel disgruntled all evening . . . until he discovered that the very plane he'd missed had crashed. There were no survivors. Paul's irritation swiftly shifted to gratitude, as he acknowledged that the unexpected change of plans had spared his life.

Change can do funny things to people and their attitudes. One time, when I was moving to a new home, I excitedly told my friends, "This move will be great! I'm letting go of a lot of stuff that no longer fits my life—it will be a welcome change!" This comment was met with gloomy warnings and associations of change with death and taxes. In that moment, I realized that I had a choice: to be influenced by outside opinions, embrace struggle, and delay my happiness *or* to be open and celebrate the change.

> *"This being human is a guest house.*
> *Every morning a new arrival.*
> *A joy, a depression, a meanness,*
> *some momentary awareness comes*
> *as an unexpected visitor.*
> *Welcome and entertain them all!"*

— **Rumi** (translated by Coleman Barks)

One morning, my friend and I went on a walk in the mountains. As the sun was rising, it looked like an egg yolk resting perfectly inside a round hole at the top of the highest peak of the mountain. It was breathtaking. We stood still in silent amazement.

Early the next morning, with camera in hand, I traveled to the exact same spot . . . only to find there was no sunrise. Clouds were blocking its majesty. Years have gone by, and I've never again seen the sun rest atop the crater at the mountain's peak.

The lesson I received from Mother Nature was a simple one: Nature is all about change, and if we hold on to what has already been, lamenting and resisting its loss, we might miss the next spectacular event. To understand how the natural world responds to change so gracefully and effortlessly, we can look at how the day is constantly shifting: from the rising of the sun in the east to bright high noon, to the colorful sun setting in the west, and finally ending with the blackness of night.

We can also observe the changing seasons. For example, as autumn fades into winter, how does this affect the animals? Do birds give each other foreboding warnings about moving south? Do bears stress out about their impending hibernation? Do they get upset with a change of plans, second-guess themselves, or ask their animal friends what they think? No. Animals prepare for harsh conditions, follow their instincts, and quickly adapt.

The creatures of the wild adapt far more quickly and easily than humans. Farmers shake their heads at the insecticides that worked perfectly last year but are worthless this year. Doctors do the same thing with bacteria that outsmart our antibiotics. It's not likely these creatures, when faced with life and death, are saying to each other, "I just don't do well with change!" They don't try to *think-think-think* their way out of challenges, ruminating on how it shouldn't be happening this way or getting stuck on how things were so much better before. Instead, they move forward by acting upon their innate wisdom and inner guidance.

Many species will also change their natural coloring to blend in with the environment, while others are known to play dead to fool predators. An octopus can morph into the scenery by changing its skin, texture, and color, generating its own camouflage to become invisible to predators. The forces of Nature that whisper to the octopus are active in you, too. You know those gut feelings you have from time to time? You can tap into your body's innate wisdom in the same way that Nature does to successfully adapt to change.

Here's a way to turn up the volume on your inner wisdom and connection to yourself. Tune in to how your body feels when you're making decisions about change. Become still and breathe to come to a place of neutrality. Then imagine the scenarios you're trying to decide between. If your body feels tight and constricted, the decision most likely won't be as favorable as when your body feels open and expansive.

Through this contemplation in your heart, you'll receive the courage, guided by your inner knowing, to take correct action. And when you do so, a whole new positive journey is sparked. Change can be your greatest teacher, demonstrating that resistance, fear, and avoidance are barriers that block your empowerment and transformation.

Nature's Lesson #1:
Start with Very Small Changes

After several years, I visited my childhood home and was amazed by the growth of the trees. Living there, I didn't notice their changes, but coming back, I realized how Nature continues to subtly grow and evolve, maximizing personal efficiency by making small, continuous improvements, bit by bit, day by day. Over time, a masterpiece is created.

A huge task can seem overwhelming, but when you break it down into tiny increments, your brain relaxes and becomes creative. You think, *Oh, that little part is simple. I can do that!* Many people say that this is the easiest way to approach change. For example, when moving, focus on one box at a time; for a stack of paperwork, focus on one paper at a time. It's like the quote: "The man who removes a mountain begins by carrying away small stones."

Have you ever considered being comfortable with being *uncomfortable?* You can help yourself become more at ease with the unfamiliar by making small, insignificant changes in your daily routine. Here are some examples: sleeping on the opposite side of the bed, shifting your toothbrush to the other side of the sink, eating in a different chair, or taking a different route to work. Even these seemingly inconsequential steps can break your habitual patterns and mechanical ways of doing, thinking, and not noticing. They pull you out of those rigid mental grooves to allow more flexible ways of thinking.

Nature's Lesson #2:
Reside in the Eye of the Changing Storm

Another way to look at what Mother Nature does when dealing with change is to note that even in the middle of a storm, she is calm. How can you emulate this and remain calm when you're caught in a raging storm? It's possible! Think of Captain "Sully" Sullenberger, the US Airways pilot who landed his plane on the Hudson River after it hit a flock of geese and the engine failed. He was so calm during that crisis. Listening to the replay of him communicating with air-traffic control was nothing but astonishing. His ability to remain calm and focused saved lives.

Fortunately, the majority of us don't experience such extreme circumstances, but even small, everyday changes can be challenging. Personal growth and development consultant Roger B. Lane, Ph.D., the founder and director of Cosmos Tree, teaches that we're quite literally stressed *out* because we've placed most of our emphasis *out*side of ourselves.

Meditation teacher Reverend Rebecca Underwood, who studied under Roger Lane, elaborates on this notion: "We can choose to be 'de-stressed' through meditation, when we go within to our rich inner world, where the outer reference points fall away." Meditation, according to Underwood, can transport us to the eye of the ever-changing storm, which can be uncomfortable at first. She adds, "Two minutes of sitting still was as troublesome as having unnecessary dental surgery. Now, after consistent practice, I look forward to meditating and find it as satisfying as sinking into a hot mineral bath."

Underwood teaches that whenever life feels difficult, take a moment to tell yourself that you're okay. Say phrases such as: *I'm okay. I'm safe. I have everything I need. Things are fine. I'm here now. I can handle this. I'm resourceful.* She explains that even though this technique is simple, even rudimentary, the effectiveness is exponential. Self-talk can calm a racing mind, bring you back to the here-and-now, and just help take the edge off. Consider the spirit in which you approach this as well. Remember, Nature doesn't look too serious when you notice the flowers dancing in the wind.

Mother Nature can be your greatest teacher. Could you emulate the ways in which she grows and adapts? Can you embrace the mystery and magic that is life? Are you willing to find the calm in the storm and trust in the changes that happen outside of your control? Are there any other lessons on change and resilience that you can learn from Nature? Say it with me: "I do well with change!"

Another reason why many of us dislike change is because we're afraid of something bad happening. And we sometimes avoid the natural world because it can be unpredictable and, at times, a little scary. Sadly, this often prevents us from learning Nature's valuable lessons about fear and the dark side of life.

> *"It is not the strongest of the species that survive, not the most intelligent, but the one most responsive to change."*
>
> **— Charles Darwin**

> *"Life is not about waiting for the storm to pass, it's about learning to dance in the rain."*
>
> **— Anonymous**

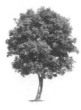

CHAPTER TWELVE

The Dark Side of Nature

"Just as the tumultuous chaos of a thunderstorm brings a nurturing rain that allows life to flourish, so too in human affairs times of advancement are preceded by times of disorder. Success comes to those who can weather the storm."

— **I Ching, No. 3**

Imagine going on a Nature walk in picture-postcard scenery with an intimate group of friends. Away from cell phones, bills, work, and pressure, you're happily trekking in the clean, fresh air of the great outdoors, surrounded by sweet-smelling flowers, deeply rooted trees, and perhaps even a fluffy bunny or two. *Ah, that sounds relaxing!*

Now imagine that you're on a different path on that Nature walk, sloshing through mud on a humid, gloomy day, with insects buzzing around your head. A hawk swoops down on that adorable little bunny, which shrieks its cry of death as the hawk's claws sink into its flesh. *Not so relaxing!*

You—Unplugged

Stephen Harper is a wilderness guide and author who leads groups of people on life-transforming experiences through his hiking workshops and retreats. At the end of a trip, his clients return home with renewed insight and hearts full of love and peace. However, the adventure is not all rosy. Some of people's greatest transformations occur in the wild, where they have less control.

Harper describes why it's important to explore the full spectrum of Nature—the dark side as well as the sunny side:

> Above all, I try to make the experience whole and honest. . . . Wilderness includes mud, gray rainy days, animal-fouled water, dark and perilous forests, and deathly dangers. Take for an example the literal and metaphoric instance of mud and rain. Our culture constantly avoids mud and rain; vacation ads depict white clean beaches and sunny skies. When it rains, everyone scampers about crouched over as though water will dissolve them like Oz's Wicked Witch of the West.
>
> Our willingness to be in the mud and rain can reflect our willingness to be in our internal mud and rain. To be "in" mud and rain is more than just tolerance; it is awareness and sometimes active participation with our own "raininess" or "muddiness." True contact with wilderness requires more than just tolerance of muddy times. Wild nature requires nothing less than attentiveness to all that is if we desire to know its secrets. This is not to advocate looking for mud puddles, or taking vacations in rainy places, although at times that may not be a bad idea. I do advocate a willingness to be with and at times to become our dark, sometimes muddy, sometimes painful, wild nature.[1]

One of Harper's guiding principles comes from Richard Price, the co-founder of the Esalen Institute in Big Sur: "Trust process, support process, and get out of the way" is demonstrated throughout Harper's expeditions. For example, he recounts the story of Marcie, a client who went on one of his trips as a getaway, a break from dealing with the newly empty nest in her life. At one point in the hike, she'd fallen behind in the group, and when Harper went back to get her, he found her standing on the trail, overwhelmed by fear:

> She was shaking uncontrollably, gasping for shallow breaths yet frozen in place. Overwhelmed with fear of falling off the trail, she was what climbers call "gripped." While the hillside we stood on was steep . . . it was far from dangerous. Earlier in my career, I would have tried to logically talk Marcie out of her fear (as though fear is logical) or I might have challenged her to be strong and overcome it.
>
> Instead, I supported her state with simply saying, "You're OK, let this happen." She burst into tears and began to shake even more. I encouraged her to allow the fear she was feeling rather than push it away.
>
> After some minutes of deep sobbing . . . she began to relate to the larger fear of feeling as though she was falling from the trail of the life she had known for so many years. Who was she, if not a mother with children to take care of? Once again, I encouraged her to enter into those feelings. After some time and more tears, Marcie began to feel the earth beneath her feet, that indeed she was being supported by the trail. That gravity was holding her to the earth more than it was pulling her off. Slowly she shifted to seeing and feeling what was there rather than what was not or no longer there.
>
> Gradually Marcie began hiking up the trail to re-join our well-rested group, with a feeling of ease and trust in her body.[1]

Harper takes groups into the wilderness so that a person can learn to face his or her shadow. Marcie was able to move through her fear by reconnecting with the earth and feeling its support. This is actually a timeworn tradition. In many cultures, ritual dances with masks and costumes, which are often conducted outdoors and depict elements of Nature, help people overcome personal trauma and difficult feelings.

Just-for-Fun Quiz!

Test Your Nature IQ!

1. Which is more dangerous: the wilderness or a city?

2. Are your chances of getting killed greater by a domestic dog or by an animal in the wild?

3. Do wolves attack humans?

Answers

1. A city is statistically more dangerous than the wilderness.

2. Domestic dogs kill more people than wild animals do.

3. It's rare for wolves to attack and kill humans.

How dangerous do you think it is to go into the wild? Harper explains that in Nature, we imagine that we're in far greater danger than we really are. Our mind can trick us when there's no threat at all. Movies that portray ferocious wolves are deceiving because in reality, wolves are rarely known to attack people. It's also uncommon for a mountain lion to attack a human. In fact, since 1990, they've only killed ten people in the U.S. and Canada.

Scientist Tom Chester recounts that in the U.S., between 1979 and the late 1990s, domestic dogs have killed more than 300 people. According to Chester, "This means that your family dog or your neighbor's dog is ten times more likely to kill you than is a mountain lion and hundreds of times more likely than a coyote."[2] Statistically, the "urban jungle" is more dangerous than being out in the "wild." Of course, it's wise to always be aware of your surroundings no matter where you are.

If Every Day Were Sunny . . .

In our culture, we're constantly sold the idea that we should avoid anything unpleasant or uncomfortable. But what would our lives be like without the dark side, which helps us to appreciate the light and the good?

There's a TV episode that begins with a gangster being gunned down. It then cuts to him waking up in a mansion with servants all around. He opens a closet to find an elaborate wardrobe designed just for him. Gourmet meals are prepared for him. Many series of events happen and they all go his way. He has everything.

After months and months of absolutely no problems and everything going perfectly, he starts a game of pool and with one shot, all the balls go into the pockets. He turns and barks to one of his servants, "If this is heaven, I'd rather be in hell!"

The servant replies, "That's where you are."

Our life challenges can seem to be rainy, muddy, and filled with pests, but we act as if that were unnatural. We complain about our hardships and identify with them, defining our life by their ebb and flow. We forget that rainy days are part of Nature, too. Nature welcomes fierce storms, surprising events, and harsh conditions.

Professors Ron Hulnick, Ph.D., and Mary Hulnick, Ph.D., teach us that how we relate to the issue *is* the issue. And as Viktor Frankl, who survived the concentration camps during the Holocaust, eloquently states of his experience: "Between stimulus and response there is a space. In that space is the power to choose our response. In our response lies our growth and freedom." He also suggests that we decide what we wish to be "in spite of conditions."

What would it be like to roll with our rainy, muddy, pest-filled days, rather than cursing the "bad" weather? Could we simply attend to stormy weather, without all the drama? Once again, let's look to Nature, who is flexible and flourishes despite the dark, harsh aspects. Seemingly severe events like a thunderstorm, a forest fire, a predator killing a small animal, or even the contrast between the eye of the hurricane and the raging winds that surround it, teach us about the relationship between darkness and light.

You can get through many challenges, knowing that no matter how difficult they may seem, they're a natural part of life. It's never always sunny in Nature—cloudy days happen and storms threaten. Remember that rainy days nourish future growth.

> ### Nature's Secret Message
> **Without the intense heat of forest fires (caused naturally by lightning), certain species of pinecones can't open to release their seeds so new pines can grow. Hidden in what seem like adversities are often divine whispers of blessings and (quite literally) opportunities for growth.**

Finding the Blessings

What if the universe were conspiring for your good? Remember that Nature's fires spark new development. Can you recall events in your life that seemed terrible at the time but ended up working toward your benefit? Now think of any present difficulties you're experiencing and see if you can uncover their hidden blessings. Fill in the blanks in the following sentences to help you get started:

Because I _____ [describe a past difficult experience or troubling feelings], *I now* _____ [describe how it transformed into a blessing].

Because I _____ [fill in a present event or situation that distresses you], *I will* _____ [think of ways this "negative" can serve as a positive experience for your own growth].

Whenever you feel stressed, could you look at what blessing the universe may be giving you in the situation? I know it can be challenging, but keep in mind that this experience may help you uncover your unused talents and strengths. In the words of Rainer Maria Rilke: "Allow life to happen to you. Believe me, life is right in all cases."

Observing Your Issues for Answers

Herbalists observe a plant's characteristics to discover its benefits. They study everything about the plant: its roots, stems, leaves, flowers, location, actions, fruits, and soil. For example, they might note that if a plant grew in an environment where there was little accessible water, it would have an adequate ability to conserve water.

What if you observed all the aspects of an issue that you're facing in the same way in which herbalists observe every aspect of the plants they study? What are the "roots" of your situation? What "fruit" is it giving you? In what "soil" do you mentally plant your thoughts? Can you have compassion for the storms within you?

"Healing is the flooding with loving to the places inside that hurt or suffer, thereby dissolving them."

— **Drs. Ron** and **Mary Hulnick**

"Everything has its wonders, even darkness and silence, and I learn, whatever state I may be in, therin to be content."

— **Helen Keller**

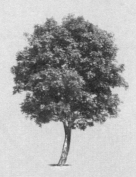

Part IV

Nature's Secrets about
Food, Drugs, and Deception

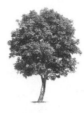

CHAPTER THIRTEEN

The Ugly Side of Beauty

*"Although human subtlety makes a variety of inventions . . .
it will never devise an invention more beautiful, more simple,
or more direct than does nature, because in her inventions
nothing is lacking, and nothing is superfluous."*

— **Leonardo da Vinci**

As we've discussed throughout this book, to truly understand and benefit from the secrets that Nature is so eager to share with us, we have to be willing to see with new eyes. This requires looking at the whole picture—rather than just what we see on the surface.

Let's traipse down to the produce department to discover more secrets that are hidden in plain sight. See the lovely fruit and vegetables lined up just so? They may look appealing at first, but think about it for a moment . . . do they really look like that in Nature? Our society's obsession with beauty (which includes our fascination with plastic-surgery-sculpted celebrities) has blinded us to yet another of Nature's secrets: *There's perfection in imperfection.*

Groceries Going Hollywood

The grocery store's produce section is like an Academy Awards party—a glitzy-looking group of fruits and vegetables that clean up very well. These are the "star" foods that made the cut, appearing at a supermarket near you.

Oh, look—the flawless, model oranges are posing! The scarlet apples look lip-glossed. I wonder what wax they're wearing? Who helped those voluptuous pears fit so perfectly into their containers? The peaches have such creamy skin, not a blemish in sight. The rack of melons seems so plump that I wonder if they're real. The "baby" carrots are trimmed down and cleaned up, their line-free skin looking positively Botoxed. Larger, perfectly erect carrots look ready for action. And then there are the international stars, a global mix of polished fruits and veggies from halfway around the world, including the spectacularly symmetrical kiwis sporting expensive price tags.

Wow! All these stand ready for their close-up inspection by the grocery shoppers. *Ah!* They're the winners . . . right? On the other hand, perhaps like the Hollywood stars who've been nipped, Photoshopped, and professionally made up, this star-level produce isn't what it appears to be.

I used to select only the most beautiful produce—yes, I wanted the best! Don't we all? But what's the cost of this obsession with appearance? Attention shoppers! The specials may not be so special!

Could we be buying with our eyes but missing out on things like . . . well, let's see . . . enjoying rich flavors and high nutritional values, helping needy people, maintaining sustainability and a healthy environment, and respecting the planet? Let's look at the *gross* in grocery produce.

Stepford Chives: "Perfect,"
Identical Fruits and Vegetables

Have you ever wondered how most grocery produce is uniform in size and color—and manage to slip into their perfect-sized containers? What tree in Nature grows only ideal fruit of the same size and shape? Since when does Nature produce only uniform, flawless food?

"Grocery-store produce is so perfect—it's not perfect," concludes farmer Gene Etheridge of Etheridge Organic Fruit and Citrus Farms.[1] What he means is that *natural food is imperfect!* Nature creates food in all sizes and shapes, some with flaws, and numerous variations. Yet in the grocery stores, we're seeking standardized beauty.

Early one morning in a local supermarket, I watched some of the tomatoes being neatly lined up. There was the produce guy, like *American Idol* star Simon Cowell, sizing up the veggies, picking the prettiest ones, and tossing the rest into a cardboard box for disposal. Those had made it past several inspections, but they didn't make it into the finals.

A few days later, I was in another store where the produce guy (I'll call him "Juan"; he prefers to be anonymous) was also tossing food into cardboard boxes. Curious, I asked what he was doing, and he said that he was instructed to throw out anything that didn't look good and to trim any "defects." (A defect is anything that makes the produce look "homely.")

I asked if the food in the "reject" box was still good. "Of course. Sometimes we'll cut up the fruit and sell it in to-go containers, but if we left the bruised fruit on the shelf, it wouldn't sell. You can juice these carrots, and use those tomatoes for a tasty sauce," he said, pointing to the growing pile in the discard box.

"Why not sell the 'uglies' for half price, rather than throw them out?" I asked.

"The store tried it, but it doesn't work. People think there's something wrong with it, even though there isn't."

"Why not give it to homeless or starving people who could use the food?"

"We've been given firm orders to throw the food out—even the employees can't take any home," Juan replied.

The garbage containers at the store are actually locked away, so I couldn't get a photo. Juan told me that he could lose his job if he took a picture of the private garbage. He claimed that the store worries about lawsuits and feels pressure to comply with FDA rules, so it all gets locked up and tossed out.

When I said it was wasteful to throw it out, he responded, "If you think this is bad, go to downtown Los Angeles, where wholesalers sell the food to stores. You'll be amazed by all the food that's thrown out because it doesn't *look* good—there are Dumpsters full."

Like a barber snipping away unwanted ends, he continued, saying, "Where I'm from in Mexico, we're poor, so we use *all* the food. We can't afford to just throw away something because it doesn't look good. In America, most people buy with their eyes and waste a lot. Children at my son's school take one bite of their lunch and throw the rest away." In other parts of the world, this would be unheard of.

I visited another grocery store and found a similar scenario. The produce worker was unpacking fresh food that had just arrived. His job is called "cleaning," which means getting rid of any flaws. He began tearing the outer leaves off the cabbages, tossing them in a box with the bent celery. He told me that he knows the food is perfectly good but won't sell the way it is, so he keeps cutting and peeling away. "The wrinkled tangerines are so much sweeter," he remarked, "but they won't sell because they're not pretty."

He told me that his store composts the rejected food, minimizing waste and ensuring that our future soil is healthier. Other stores don't want to bother with any form of recycling, though; they simply throw out all the rejects. In Nature, there is little or no waste, but we waste food simply because it's not aesthetically pleasing.

A friend who works at a TV studio tells me that the amount of food that's wasted on sets is shocking, saying the cooks feed the crew and sometimes have 30 or 40 burgers left over that get tossed. Likewise, in his book *The Omnivore's Dilemma,* Michael Pollan writes that Native Americans felt corn was sacred and would be astonished and disheartened to see modern farms leave spilled corn scattered all over the place, wasted and disregarded.

As I was reading more about Native Americans and early settlers, and their arduous struggles to find food under extreme weather conditions to survive, I became immersed in their plight. Think of how much you would appreciate food if you had just survived a famine or a blizzard! I understood why they held food as sacred—to them, it was a gift from the heavens. Native Americans felt that eating was like making love with the planet. After consuming their food, they'd be sure to plant a seed back into the soil to show respect and gratitude.

While reading about these rituals, I lost track of time; it grew late and I was hungry. I braved the cold for a few minutes to get to my heated car to drive to the grocery store just a few blocks away. As I entered the supersized store, the bright lights and colors stopped me in my tracks. I was taken aback by the excessive abundance. I stood staring at all the washed, cleaned, and cooked food, ready for my selection. It was such an extreme display of food that I actually felt stunned and dismayed that night. I wondered what it would be like for one of my ancestors to see this loaded supermarket, then to witness the imperfect food being tossed in the garbage to rot.

That same week, I watched a video on how we need to make *more* food for starving people. I couldn't help thinking, *But what about the enormous amount of good food in farms, stores, homes, restaurants, businesses, and schools that we're throwing out each day?!* The Environmental News Service reports that *half* of the food produced worldwide is wasted. That means we're also wasting the water it took to grow the food. It's like the saying: "It's not how much you make, but how you manage the money." How are we managing our food resources?

That reminded me of crates and crates worth of scratched oranges left on paths to eliminate dust. Yes, tractors actually roll over all of this good food to juice the dirt paths to prevent dust flying into the trees. Farmer Gene Etheridge showed me a perfectly good orange that was scratched and informed me that if it were from a typical farm, it wouldn't make the grade and would be left on the ground.

Other imperfect produce is often sold at farmers' markets. What's the difference between the two? Are the stores getting the "stars," while the duds hit the outdoor markets? And if our food is so great, then why is our society riddled with obesity and diabetes? I went to my local farmers' market to find answers.

Food— a Premature Birth?

Modern society has a way of rushing food before it's fully ripened. If a woman told you she was pregnant and wanted to force her baby to be born much earlier because she's busy, you might think that's not such a good idea for the baby's health. Obviously, the unborn child needs time to develop to full-term.

It's similar with produce selected for stores. When the fruit and vegetables are picked on time, we get the full nutritional value, but the store takes on more risk of spoilage. On the other hand, produce picked prematurely has a longer shelf life. A farmer even told me that most stores only want to buy rock-hard avocados since they have more "staying power."

This is another reason why farmers' markets selling local produce are better: the food is allowed to grow until it's ripe, delivering more nutrients *and* better taste—which is highly beautiful to me, even though it doesn't look perfect.

"Casual Friday" for Produce?

Sunny Santa Monica, California, is known for its Wednesday morning farmers' market. Blocks of stalls with fruits and veggies in all sizes and shapes are thrown together in boxes, quite unlike the glitzy grocery-store displays. Here, the food has flaws and dirt, and many can't fit into those perfect little containers. Is it "casual Friday" for produce?

My first purchase is organic corn. The farmer nonchalantly asks, "You want me to take the caterpillar off the corn?" as if it's routine to have a bug crawling on my food.

"Excuse me?"

She casually peels away the top part of the corn's husk, exposing a caterpillar and removing the wiggly worm. If a caterpillar is discovered at a store, there would probably be complaints—but I guess it's common at this stand.

I mosey around, rummaging through a big box of oranges, kind of like shopping at discount stores, looking for the good stuff. I see oranges with shades of green, dirt, wrinkles, and scratches. Thinking these oranges are inferior, I'm about to leave when the farmer notices me. He explains that the green shading means that it's the second picking, so they're the sweetest, juiciest oranges I'll ever eat. The green actually comes from the way these late-season oranges "regreen" to protect themselves from the abundance of sunshine, which causes chlorophyll to collect on the rind. He offers me a sample to see for myself. Juice squirts in my mouth. *Wow!* Now, that's an orange. It's one of the best-tasting, juiciest, greenest, and "ugliest" oranges I ever ate. I enthusiastically buy several dirty, multicolored, scratched, and scuffed oranges.

Another farmer tells me that it's difficult to sell good food to retailers unless it looks pretty. He mentions several companies that will only buy pretty fruit, which ultimately means using more insecticides to keep bugs from scarring it. Fruit gets softer later in the season, and when they're packed tight, they dimple, but this also indicates that they're sweeter, too. External thrips scars, sharpshooter and spittle, or katydid bites (I guess that's farmers' lingo for imperfections caused by insects!) are just proof that insecticides were *not* used. It's the inside—where the taste and nourishment are—that counts!

"Try a visually distressed fruit," the farmer offers. "I think you'll find it to be just as tasty, if not tastier, than the pretty stuff."

I taste. As my mouth salivates, I feel like those people on Sunday-morning TV who proclaim, "Hallelujah—I've seen the light!" As a customer next to me bags her produce, she says with passion, "I come here because I feel like I'm close to 'the source,' choosing from the freshest food, rather than food picked way too early just for an extended shelf life in the stores." *Another convert.*

A few feet away another customer, a self-proclaimed foodie, pipes in and says that those huge strawberries at supermarkets have no taste and are bred to be large for chocolate dipping, which *looks* great. He instructs me to pick up some freshly picked strawberries here because they taste like . . . well, like *real* strawberries!

I move on to another huge block of produce. As I'm selecting dirty, crooked carrots, I overhear someone raving about blue eggs. This radiant, healthy-looking woman turns to me (or really, to anyone who will listen) and proclaims, "The free-range eggs in the store are a joke! This man's chickens are roaming around happy, with space and open air like they're supposed to be raised—rather than all cooped up or given a mere few feet to 'roam.' You can taste a huge difference. Do a taste test for yourself—and they're so much better for you!"

Okay. She sold me. I tell the farmer I'll buy his eggs. "Nope, ya can't," he says, as if he couldn't care less if he makes the sale or not. "They're all sold out." I'll need to get to the market earlier next time if I want the coveted blue eggs. So I buy my dirty carrots and move to the next booth, now lusting for the eggs I can't have.

I walk over to a farmer who appears to be in his mid-70s. His hands shake visibly as he proudly shows me his organic dried herbs, like a jeweler who exhibits rare gems. I notice that he's under a tent with a wide variety of products on his stand and truck. He's working hard; he needs to set up, sell, take down, and pack everything back up all by himself. I buy several herbs to jazz up the taste of my dishes, and to support this humble man.

As I amble through the market, I hear an exclamation: "Oh, wow—you have *raw dates!*" A man turns to me, saying, "You gotta try these." He's not even with the farm stand, just a date enthusiast. But they don't even look like dates since they're sold in clusters on thin beige vines. I taste one and *ooohhh*—they're really yummy and not too sweet. I don't particularly like dates, but these raw ones are amazingly tasty so I buy a few strands.

"Would you like to try a barbecued plum?" A vibrant-looking farmer is serving up samples in the next booth. He explains that if I cook these plums with fish or chicken, they'll caramelize the food, giving it a wonderful taste. I try one. *Mmm, it tastes like candy.*

I haul my loot to the car. Feeling hungry, I grab an orange and peel its imperfect skin. What the heck is this? The amount of juice that comes gushing out astounds me. I hit a geyser! It's like someone poured juice into my orange. I'd never seen *this* with a grocery-store orange. And my peaches are so juicy that I have to eat them over the sink!

Those herbs really do spice up my food, and the not-sweet dates become my favorite crunchy snack—similar to the crunch you get from water chestnuts. I can eat 'em like chips and immediately wished I bought more.

Two weeks later, I return to feed my new addiction. Running up to the date stand, I say, "I want to purchase a lot of your yummy raw dates! They're my favorite snack, I—"

The farmer interrupts, saying, "It's past the season, and they're all gone." For a minute, I'm like a kid on Christmas day who discovered there's no fire engine under the tree. However, this experience gave me another lesson from Nature. I now look forward to the time when those crunchy raw dates will be in season again.

My friend Robin, who grew up in California, told me she knew the seasons by which foods were growing. What a delightful experience for her when juicy peaches were in season! Could having a cornucopia of foods from all over the world, so readily accessible, kind of cheapen the glory of seasonal fruit? *Oh yeah, a peach—I can get that anytime.*

Now I understand why the customer was sharing his excitement about raw dates with everyone. You *can't* get them whenever you want. I'm sure when I see raw dates again, I'll be just as enthused and ready to proclaim to anyone around: "You gotta try these!" Would I do that if I could get them all the time? Probably not. I have a feeling that each season is going to be like rekindling an old love.

Mother Nature teaches us to appreciate what we have *now*, and to look forward to the gifts she gives us in the upcoming seasons. By growing organic fruits and vegetables and eating locally, we're slowly but surely counteracting the damage we've done to the soil and environment, and we're learning to pace and protect our productivity while also supporting our local farmers.

Nature's Secret Message

Nature's bounty in all sizes and shapes is the real thing, signaling that beauty, power, and value lie beneath the surface. Just because a fruit or vegetable looks imperfect, it doesn't mean that it's any less nutritious. In fact, it might even taste *better!*

Permaculture—Taking Nature Off Our Leash

I visited gardener Jeanette Aguilar's home in Los Angeles to learn about permaculture, a culture of living sustainably by growing your own food, building natural homes, establishing eco-communities, and much more. In fact, the international environmental advocate David Suzuki asserts: "What permaculturists are doing is the most important activity that any group is doing on the planet."

Jeanette teaches companies to grow on-site organic gardens that fill their cafeterias with healthy, nutritious food, while at the same time helping to "regreen" the environment. "If every corporation grew a garden, more oxygen would be generated into our cities," she explains. "If every corporation educated people on how to grow food in their own backyards or on balconies, we would all be doing our small part, helping to create food for our families and sharing it with communities that need it."

As we stepped into Jeanette's kitchen, she offered me yogi tea made from scratch (which included cloves, cardamom pods, black peppercorns, cinnamon, gingerroot, black tea, purified water, and fragrant edible flowers). It was already brewing on the stove, and next to it simmered homemade mung-bean soup.

With tea in hand, we strolled out to her small backyard, and I felt like I'd stepped into a little piece of paradise. Strawberries, celery, kale, Swiss chard, cauliflower, tomatoes, raspberries, and eggplant all greeted me. Her garden isn't arranged in straight rows, either, but in swirls. This made a lot of sense to me, as Nature generally moves in waves and circles. Why not plant that way? If you look at the garden at **www.perelandra-ltd.com**, you'll see that it grows in the shape of phi—a swirl.

In one corner of the garden are colorful, edible flowers: nasturtium and calendula that she adds to her salads, turning them into works of art. Herbs grow here, too, including basil, lemon thyme, oregano, parsley, lemongrass, and rosemary; and a variety of fruit trees overlook the yard, such as satsuma tangerine, Meyer lemon, loquat, banana, mango, Asian pear, and Hass avocado. Tropical orchids, bromeliads, succulents, annuals, and perennials add even more color and beauty. As we toured her intimate garden, she told me that it constantly evolves. She had plans to grow corn, squash, beans, a variety of peppers, and much more in the summer.

To water her garden, Jeanette relies on a gray-water system that reuses dish, shower, sink, and laundry wastewater (but none from toilets). This is a perfect way to reuse that water without wasting it or incurring the expense of treatment. She also puts grass clippings and dried leaves back onto the soil, which creates a mulch that holds the moisture in the soil after watering. It's kind of like giving the earth an extra blanket that acts as a barrier to the evaporation process. The soil stays moist longer and needs less watering than if it were not covered up. This is a beautiful act, but it isn't as manicured, or as some might think, beautiful looking.

(You may not want to grow all of your own food, but it's not difficult to grow at least some of it. And every little bit is a step forward. For tips on how to easily start an organic garden, see Appendix I.)

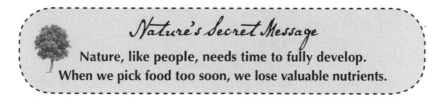

Nature's Secret Message
Nature, like people, needs time to fully develop.
When we pick food too soon, we lose valuable nutrients.

Lookin' Good—at What Cost?

One farmer shared his dirty secrets about "ugly" food with me. He told me that the *uglies* (those with wind or insect scars; or that are puffy, creased, or generally unattractive) will go directly to the juice market, which usually doesn't pay enough to offset production costs. If the fruit grown isn't enough to get top dollar, they may as well tear out the trees and put in row crops, or sell the land to a developer for homes or shopping malls.

Unfortunately, many beautiful, fruitful orange groves are being ripped out because of increasing costs and because so much of our fruit now comes from other countries.

The farmer I spoke with sums up the situation: "Some orange companies have a marketing philosophy that their name can only be used on the 'prettiest' fruits. Ultimately, farmers lose out from not being able to market good fruit at the best price possible, and that's a big reason you see orange groves being pushed out. Most fruit—plus or minus 50 to 60 percent—is considered visually distressed in one way or another. This cavalier grading system causes producers to lean toward pesticides to reduce what is just superficial insect scarring.

"Early-picked fruit generally is the prettiest, but it often has a lower sugar-to-acid ratio," he added. "Growers lose fair market prices when their fruits get rejected by the juice marketers. Oranges may be sweeter after the trees sit through the summer."

Nature's Secret Message

**Nature's perfection lies
within our perceived imperfection.**

Beautiful, Convenient Carrots

A high-tech carrot farm has a camera that can detect carrots that aren't perfectly sized and a machine that can quickly reject misshapen ones. Stores won't take perfectly good food that's the "wrong" shape. The farmer of the site brags, "Yep, our carrots are grown in sand so we can get them perfectly straight!" When I asked him what the nutritional difference was between soil-grown and sand-grown carrots, he sounded perplexed. "What? We've never been asked that," he replied. "Uh . . . I have no idea."

What about those minicarrots that are cleaned, cut, peeled, and packaged for us? They're beautiful, but according to "Mr. Carrot," John Stolarczyk, curator of the World Carrot Museum, the best nutrition is just beneath the skin; and peeling removes 15 percent of the carotene—along with some trace minerals. He adds that "baby" carrots are "shaved and abrasively tumbled," and therefore aren't as healthy as whole carrots. The majority of the goodness is in or just under the skin, as it is with most fruit and vegetables. As you get closer to the center, the nutritional goodness decreases.[2]

Many packages of carrots don't list the amount of beta-carotene and vitamin C content. Yet according to the USDA, 100 grams of raw carrots have 8,285 mcg of beta-carotene and 5.9 mg of vitamin C. The same volume of baby carrots has only 6,391 mcg of beta-carotene and 2.6 mg of vitamin C. Mr. Carrot sums it up this way: "There's a third less beta-carotene in baby-cut carrots and two-thirds less vitamin C. But there are high profits in baby carrots. Look at the weight-for-weight price. The farmers tell me that supermarkets demand carrots that look nice in the packets and don't mention anything about nutritional value to the grower. It's all down to price and looks."[2]

Here's the bottom line on cut, shaved, and cleaned carrots: yes, they're more convenient and they're better than not eating any vegetables . . . but the carrots you wash and cut yourself have more nutritional value and are less expensive.

Apple "Makeup"

Remember those shiny apples that look like they're wearing lip gloss? A government scientist who specializes in fruit waxes told me that this process makes fruit look shiny but slightly alters the taste. Some wax ingredients are proprietary but have to be made from ingredients approved by the FDA. However, it's hard for the FDA to keep current with the deluge of information as to any ill effects. Why can't we know more about what's been done to our food, especially since it's been shown that certain waxes affect the taste?

Store owners may gloss over the differences between waxed and unwaxed foods, but do we really need to "polish" apples in the first place? Just because an apple is beautiful and shiny doesn't mean it's a better choice.

Beauty and the Meats

> *"Man digs his grave with his fork and spoon."*
>
> — Anonymous

Have you ever noticed that when you're supertired, a little blush can make a big difference? It's a simplistic example, but it's similar to what's happening to our meat products, which are also being made "prettier."

You see meat in the grocery store that *looks* fresh, so it must be very fresh, right? Not necessarily. It may have been exposed to gases that make it stay red and extend its shelf life. According to the USDA: "Modified atmosphere packaging (MAP) and controlled atmosphere packaging (CAP) help to preserve foods by replacing some or all of the oxygen in the air inside the package with other gases such as carbon dioxide or nitrogen."[3] Some packagers also add carbon monoxide (CO-MAP) to their products; and as stated by the Institute of Food, Nutrition and Human Health, this enhances meat color but "CO-MAP, under certain conditions, may pose a food-safety risk."

As you may have guessed, this has stirred up much debate. One side claims that gassing meat is a safe method for preserving it, but opponents say that this is like applying makeup so the meat doesn't look as old as it is. I called a meat buyer for a large company who didn't want to be quoted, but I finally got this out of him: "We don't do it because we think it's deceiving. It keeps the meat looking red, but it could be spoiled." Some supermarket chains, such as Kroger and Publix, don't carry meat packaged with carbon monoxide. One scientist I spoke with was a strong proponent for MAP but against CO-MAP.

The July 2006 issue of *Consumer Reports* stated that for ground beef sealed in the mix of gases, shelf life could be extended "from about 14 days to 28 days, and from about 10 days to 35 days for whole cuts." In addition, they conducted testing on samples from three companies and found that the meat "appeared red even if it was spoiled or had bacterial counts that were close to indicating spoilage." Moreover, the article adds: "By their use- or freeze-by date, seven samples were fresh but two packages of ground beef from one company were spoiled; an additional sample was on the brink of spoilage a day before the stamped date."[4]

Stores also make meat look more appealing by making sure that it doesn't resemble an animal. In many cases, they cut it up, remove the bones, and package it in unrecognizable forms. When I was in Germany, pigs' heads and other distinct animal parts were commonly on display in the farmers' markets. They were selling meat that looked like animals. It was such a turnoff for me, the sheltered American: *Oh my gosh, that's a . . . dead animal! Eww, I don't want to eat that!* American grocery stores have taken Nature out of the picture . . . except in pictures.

Tantalizing Food Ads

There's an art to photographing products to enhance sales. Did you know that the majority of magazine photos are touched up in some manner? My director friend told me it's a secret that they retouched a film, frame by frame, in order to enhance the blue of the leading lady's eyes. The stylist for a photographer takes plain clothes and alters them or even pins them in back on the model to make them fit better and look more stylish than they actually are.

The same philosophy applies to food. Perfect "hero food" (an advertising-industry term) is used in commercials and print ads. A food artist makes the product appear as appetizing as possible. I've seen this several times when acting in food commercials: after each on-camera bite, I'd get another "hero food," all dressed up with perfectly placed garnishes so the product looked as beautiful as possible for the next shot. I remember seeing an entire table of "camera ready" food and watching the food stylist decorate each item with the utmost attention to detail, even using a tweezer. It's just not real, but that's what we end up believing our food *should* look like. Have you ever noticed how the tantalizing food in commercials doesn't actually look like the food you buy, because the rushed workers aren't taking their time and being paid more to make camera-ready food?

Beauty . . . at What Price?

Farmer Gene Etheridge informed me that people are often surprised to learn that kiwifruit grows in shapes other than oval. And the price we pay for this "perfect" fruit? Because there are fewer uniform kiwis, the cost goes *way* up—it's the simple law of supply and demand. I've eaten an odd-shaped kiwi and had juice rolling down into my sleeves. What a treat! I was almost giddy eating this succulent fruit at such a great price. Generally, farmers' markets not only have fresher food but better prices, too. Sometimes in stores, we're paying extra for our food to look good. Is our beautiful food having an ugly effect on our health, though?

Sour Grapes for Mother Nature—
Taking the Seeds Out of Grapes

Seeds in grapes aren't very popular, so scientists decided to improve on Mother Nature and get rid of them. Let's look at what happens when we try to "correct" Nature.

Simple logic: when scientists examine seeds, they can deduce ways in which they may help our bodies. Seeds are proactive in fighting bacteria in the plant, so it might make sense to infer that they can fight bacteria in us, too. Recent research supports this, showing that grape-seed extract contains antibacterial, antifungal, antiplatelet, and antioxidant properties. It's also a bioflavonoid, which helps strengthen blood-vessel walls. (There we go again with the grape being good for the blood!)

The highest concentration of phytochemicals is in the grape *seeds*. Grape seeds contain oligomeric proanthocyanidins (OPCs), which are among the most powerful antioxidants for preventing free-radical damage, lowering cholesterol, and improving circulation and skin elasticity. It also helps the body resist tissue deterioration, inflammation, and other oxidative damage.

The journal *Clinical Cancer Research* reports that a study at the University of Kentucky revealed that grape-seed extract helped destroy 76 percent of leukemia cells. So do we really want to take the seeds *out* of our grapes? When we tamper with Mother Nature, we may be taking a shot in the dark since there's so much more going on than we can ever imagine.

Now let's look at what we're taking out of salt. To the ancients, salt was a "media darling." Homer praised it as a "divine substance," and Jesus gave it a four-star rating, referring to his people as, "the salt of the earth, light of the world." Plato chimed in, proclaiming it as "essentially dear to the gods." Long ago, salt was even used as currency. Now, salt is the enemy—contributing to high blood pressure and heart disease. Studies prove its ill effects. So what happened? How did this sacred food shake out of favor?

We buy with our eyes. Sea salt looked dirty and clumpy. So during the industrial revolution, it received a makeover through chemical cleaning and by adding aluminum hydroxide in high heat. Oh, what a change! Now it's pure, sparkly white and pours freely—a beautiful product that will sell! But what price did we pay for meddling with this "divine substance"?

In our quest for beauty, our processing leeches out 70 to 82 elements for mineralizing the body and adds toxic chemicals that medical research has proved to be harmful. This pretty table salt is now known to produce the ugly effects of edema, cellulite, and swelling. Our ancestors—with their mineralized, *un*processed pure white salt—were right again.

> *Nature's Secret Message*
> **Salt was sacred and full of minerals until it became
> toxic when it was chemically changed to look pretty.**

A similar whitening process is also used for bread making. White bread is "dead bread," however, because the processing of the chemically bleached flour removes vitamins and minerals. It's then "enriched" with synthetic additives so that the label can say it contains vitamins! Mother Nature's message? It's not safe to rely on looks and ignore what's inside.

"Eat God-made foods, not man-made foods."

— **Dr. Khalid Mahmud**

Beautiful Solutions

You can do a number of things that will make a positive difference for your own health and well-being . . . *and* the planet's! If everyone would make even just a few small changes in the way they shop and eat, it could profoundly affect the world. Here are some truly beautiful solutions to help you get started:

— **Support local farmers and buy locally grown foods.** You'll get fresh, more nutritious produce. Sometimes food is over a week old by the time you buy it, and it's picked prematurely, which means it may be missing nutrients. Food grown locally in oxygen-generating orchards usually tastes better, too. Mother Nature gets to do her job without interference; and this also limits fuel, transportation costs, and pollution to the environment.

LocalHarvest.org offers a list of farmers in your area; and you can even buy organic, family-farmed food online. You can also subscribe to a Community Supported Agriculture (CSA) program for high-quality seasonal produce, which is a great way to support your local farmer. It's a win-win situation, according to LocalHarvest: "Farmers receive payment early in the season, which helps with the farm's cash flow [and consumers receive] ultra-fresh food, with all the flavor and vitamin benefits. [They also] get exposed to new vegetables and new ways of cooking." Forget that same ol' routine each week. The organization adds: "It's a simple enough idea, but its impact has been profound. Tens of thousands of families have joined CSAs, and in some areas of the country, there's more demand than there are CSA farms to fill it."[5]

— **Start a garden.** The best locally grown food is the food you grow yourself! No room at your place for a garden? No problem! In many cities, you can find city-funded gardens where you can rent a plot for a nominal fee. You'll belong to a community of gardeners who have a fun time "growing" together.

You can also try container gardening if you have a porch or tiny backyard. Talk to your neighbors and local farmers about what grows well and how to care for your plants by providing the right amounts of shade, water, and appropriate soil.

Why not sign up for (or request) gardening classes offered at schools, or have school food projects where classes grow food? It's a wonderful, educational experience. My six-year-old neighbor is fascinated with my sprouting plants and comes over to check the progress. He stares in wonder at the new growth.

— **Ask your grocer to sell "homely" food at lower prices.** Why not encourage your grocer to sell the less-than-gorgeous produce they're throwing out at half price with a sign explaining that the food is just as nutritious and beautiful on the inside? I'd buy flawed organic produce at half off—wouldn't you? It's a great way to eat organic food at more affordable prices.

— **Appreciate that beauty is more than skin deep.** Can we banish the myth that "imperfect" food is inferior to uniformly shaped and sized food? Let's look further than skin deep. Just like with people, can we relish the differences and appreciate those that aren't model perfect?

In challenging economic times, understanding that Nature's imperfect foods are *perfectly* edible could help lower food costs, create less waste, and may even provide better nutrition. With more education and taste tests, people would know that superficially flawed food is just as good as the beautiful food. Packers and sellers need to get the message out that visually distressed doesn't mean less sweet or less nourishing. And do they really need to wax the fruits and keep trimming the produce?

— **Don't discard the "uglies."** If your grocer won't sell flawed produce, ask the manager to consider donating the items to soup kitchens or shelters. Or at least request that they look into composting the discarded food to minimize waste and improve the soil. Remember that healthier soil means healthier people . . . and a healthier planet.

— **Insist on easy-to-understand food labels and signs.** Too often, we're kept in the dark about what happens during the processing of our food. We need shelf-help books! Some suppliers think irradiation, gassing, and waxing are safe, but I don't want that done to my food. I'd like the right to be informed if my food is wearing "makeup."

There's such little information available about how food is grown, processed, and packaged (and how prematurely it's picked), which is a huge part of the problem. The quality of the food you eat is vital; inexpensive food may be extremely expensive for your health. Consider high-quality organic food as cheap health insurance.

Find out if your grocery store stocks meats laden with carbon monoxide, and if so, buy items with a stamped sell-by date of a couple weeks away. You'll really need to use your senses, like the ancients did, since smell and taste (and your intuition) will help you determine if the meat has gone bad. Also tell the store manager that you'd love to see them go *au naturel*.

— **Eat foods in season.** In Nature, foods have their seasons. However, because produce is available from other areas and countries, we tend to eat them out of season and sacrifice nutrition and flavor.

You'll find that the vegetables and fruits that are in season are the cheapest. Generally, if produce is out of season in your area and has traveled a long distance (possibly weeks) to get to your store, it will be much more costly. You'll stretch your dollars if you buy locally grown, organic fruits and vegetables at the farmers' market that were picked at the peak of ripeness. Here's a great tip: buy more than you need and freeze the surplus, and then you'll have it on hand to enjoy. I learned this from my date experience, and now I buy these tasty treats in abundance and freeze the leftovers to snack on long after they're out of season.

— **Reevaluate your food priorities and distribution systems.** There are starving people, yet we're throwing out an excessive amount of food because it isn't beautiful or the correct size. Let's reevaluate our distribution systems (how we can curb waste, feed more, and compost) and sizing regulations (buying more imperfect sizes) to make use of all the food we produce. If we work together and express our concerns and suggestions to our elected officials, perhaps we can come up with ways to donate excess food to those who need it, minimize waste by composting or recycling, and stop throwing out perfectly good food. Now *that* would be beautiful!

❧ ❧ ❧   ❧ ❧ ❧

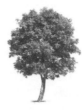

CHAPTER FOURTEEN

Prescription for Trouble

"The ark was built by amateurs.
The Titanic was built by experts."

— **Don Croft**

Pharmaceutical advertisements on TV teach us how life dramatically improves and problems disappear—all with the magic of pills. They show a depressed, shy person suddenly feeling great, dancing with a hot mate or confidently making a presentation in the boardroom. We're bombarded with images of happy, energetic people—made that way from taking pills.

We have drugs for practically everything: acid reflux, weight loss, depression, anxiety, incontinence, sexual dysfunction, and on and on. Younger women can take pills to have fewer periods, and older menopausal women can take pills to have *more* periods. Many patients expect to leave their doctor's office with a prescription in hand . . . that's the norm, right?

An article published in April 2009 in *USA Today* called "Drugs Cause Confusion in Elderly" stated that medications, both prescribed and over the counter, could impair the elderly. A patient could actually be given a wrong diagnosis because doctors don't always recognize the symptoms as a side effect of a drug.

Many prescriptions *are* necessary, but how many are *not?* And how are all these drugs affecting our bodies and the environment? Are we ignoring the serious side effects spelled out for us on the labels, which can also adversely affect the world at large? Too often, our default is to pop a pill instead of trying a natural remedy first— even though certain foods and herbs are quite often just as effective as drugs (if not more so) and don't have the nasty side effects.

Acupuncture, which originated in ancient China, is now widely used in the West as well as chiropractic, massage, Reiki, Qigong, and healing touch to activate the natural healing processes of the body and restore physical and emotional well-being. But despite their proven success, why are we reluctant to trust that we can heal ourselves without a pill?

This skewed perspective is not only further evidence of how we're out of balance with Nature, but it can also lead to our actually harming Nature. The more drugs we take, the more drugs our bodies excrete in waste, and the more they make their way into sewers and eventually into the environment. Research suggests that some of these drugs (as well as toxic substances in cleaning materials, shampoos, cosmetics, and other personal-care products) can harm fish and other animals living in our waterways.

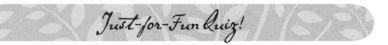

Just-for-Fun Quiz!

Test Your Nature IQ

1. *True or False:* Amounts of ibuprofen, steroids, hormones, codeine, and antibiotics have been detected in samples taken from streams throughout the United States.

2. Which of the following has *not* been used in ads that promote cigarette smoking?

   a. A baby
   b. Santa Claus
   c. A Supreme Court justice

    d. A U.S. President

    e. A pregnant woman

3. According to a BlueCross BlueShield report, how many prescription drugs does the average American take per year?

4. What place is known as the "world's lungs"?

Answers

1. True

2. A Supreme Court justice

3. 11.3

4. The rain forest is known as the world's lungs because it produces most of the available oxygen that we have.

Do we *really* know all the side effects of our drugs and the impact of combining them? In her book *Drugs: A Very Short Introduction,* Leslie Iversen discusses how it took 30 to 40 years before we could see the link between cigarette smoking and lung cancer. Some "miracle" drugs, diets, and health products were also later discovered to be dangerous and even deadly.

Or how about soldiers during World War II who liberally used DDT, thinking it would just kill mosquitoes and lice (which were carriers of typhus and malaria)? And also back then kids would run through the town sprinklers that were spraying the insecticide to decimate the mosquito population. DDT was later found to be a highly toxic carcinogen, and its use was banned in the U.S. in the early 1970s.

A recent shocking finding was in a 2008 report published in the journal *Pediatrics* regarding a new scientific detection method for hospital errors. The report notes that "medicine mix-ups, accidental overdoses, and bad drug reactions harm roughly one out of 15 hospitalized children."

> *"The US spends two times more on drugs, and*
> *takes twice as many drugs, as other countries*
> *and has worse health. That means we are paying*
> *money for drugs that aren't working for us."*

— **Doug Bremner, M.D.**

Combining Meds

Think back on all the great times you've had with your friends, just one-on-one. Now think of when you hung out with all your friends together. Did you notice that a few just don't get along?

It's the same with drugs; one on its own may be fine, but when combined with others in your body, they may not get along. Researchers have done very little testing on the effects of combining drugs and the serious complications—even death—that may follow. You can probably name several celebrities who died as a result of combining painkillers, antidepressants, and sleeping pills. But how often do you hear about celebrities overdosing on herbs?

According to a BlueCross BlueShield report, Americans take an average of 11.3 prescriptions per person per year, nationwide. That's like taking a new prescription every month! Tennessee residents lead the statistics, with 17.3 prescriptions per year for each individual, yet they're ranked 47th out of 50 in terms of health. Something isn't right.

The medical community insists a drug is safe and effective due to research, but how much research is done on the combining of many drugs? Even drinking grapefruit juice can affect how your body breaks down cholesterol-lowering drugs.

These studies can also be unreliable. *The New York Times* published a lengthy feature article in 2007 about the many ways in which clinical studies can be flawed due to bias, user compliance, atypical subjects, health of the subjects, economic status, placebo effects, faulty methodology, motivations, influences from the medical profession or those conducting the studies, statistical methods, age, timing, and the frame of mind of the people conducting and participating in the studies. Journalist Gary Taubes argues: "Observational studies can only provide what researchers call hypothesis-generating evidence—what a defense attorney would call circumstantial evidence."[1]

Sander Greenland, an epidemiologist at the University of California, Los Angeles, and author of the textbook *Modern Epidemiology,* is quoted in the *Times* article remarking that, taking all this information into account, a coin toss may be just as effective as study results. Taubes sums up the article with a quote from Elizabeth Barrett-Connor of the University of California, San Diego: "I'm back to the place where I doubt everything."[1]

She has good reason to doubt since a 2008 article in *Discover* magazine titled, "Wonder Drugs That Can Kill," reports the following:

> How often do today's medical "breakthroughs" become tomorrow's discredited science? John P. A. Ioannidis, an epidemiologist at Tufts University School of Medicine in Boston and the University of Ioannina School of Medicine in Greece, studied the question. . . . His findings, published in JAMA, show that the key claims of nearly one-third (14 out of 49) of the original research studies he examined were either false or exaggerated. Small study size, design flaws, publication bias (failure to publish negative results or duplication of positive results), drug-industry influence, and the play of chance were among the problems Ioannidis found that caused false or exaggerated claims.[2]

In the words of Karl Menninger, M.D.: "One of the most untruthful things possible, you know, is a collection of facts, because they can be made to appear so many different ways."

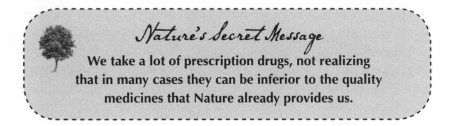

Nature's Secret Message

We take a lot of prescription drugs, not realizing that in many cases they can be inferior to the quality medicines that Nature already provides us.

Studies Create Fads

As early as the 1400s, nutrition guides were "bestsellers," giving health advice that would go in and out of popularity throughout the years. In 1933, cigarette advertisements began to appear in the *Journal of the American Medical Association.* And for eight years, the Camel cigarette slogan was: "More doctors smoke Camels than any other cigarette." In addition, doctors, babies, a pregnant woman, Santa Claus, and Ronald Reagan (who would later become President) all appeared in advertisements promoting smoking. Now it's common knowledge that cigarettes are unhealthy, and doctors today certainly don't recommend that their patients smoke. This is yet another about-face on previously established beliefs.

Margarine was initially touted as a healthy alternative to butter. However, in 1990, scientists discovered that hydrogenated oils and trans fats (also called trans-fatty acids) are linked to obesity, diabetes, high cholesterol, cancer, and heart disease. Also consider how the popular fat-free diet craze quickly faded when scientists asserted that humans need some dietary fat for the brain and body to function.

> *"Until man duplicates a blade of grass,*
> *Nature can laugh at his so-called scientific knowledge."*
>
> — **Thomas Edison**

Have you heard the story of the mother who gives her new daughter-in-law her meatball recipe? It's her son's favorite! However, she secretly leaves out a few ingredients so that the bride's recipe is lacking and the son will always miss his mama's home cooking.

In a similar manner, many drugs and supplements are attempts to re-create Mother Nature's recipes, but since we don't know all of Nature's ingredients, we don't have the complete recipe, and our attempts to produce the originals are usually lacking. Supplements and drug manufactures may chemically alter their products.

If we don't know all of the long-term effects of drugs, and we make mistakes in our studies, could we be missing some key information on the effects of medications and over-the-counter drugs on the environment? Prescription drugs are highly processed and have molecules removed so that someone can own the patent. The body doesn't know what to do with some synthetics, which are included in some supplements, too.

Mother Nature's medicine is from food, plants, and herbs. Her secrets are revealed to us through intuition and the wisdom handed down by those who have studied its medicinal properties. Unfortunately, there's less financial profit in selling the healing plants and foods of the earth than there is in selling pharmaceutical drugs. Fresh organic foods are Nature's powerful medicine! Be sure to watch the documentary *Simply Raw* (which I mentioned earlier) that shows how by simply changing their diet, several people with diabetes were able to go off all of their medications within 30 days and still maintain their blood-sugar levels. Instead of reaching into their medicine cabinet, they now look into Nature's bounty.

Nature's Secret Message

Nature provides cures we need without harming the environment.

Unintended Environmental Side Effects

When people think about pollution, most think it occurs outside of the home. However, our pharmaceuticals and personal-care products (also known as PPCPs) are now recognized as some of the most pervasive pollutants in the environment. So what are PPCPs? They include medicines such as antibiotics and birth control pills that we excrete and improperly dispose of, antimicrobial soap, shampoos, fragrances, and cleaning products that find their way into the soil and bodies of water through our wastewater and disposal systems.

Some studies show there are currently more than $70 billion worth of expired drugs in people's medicine cabinets across the United States. How will these be disposed of? It's estimated that American prescription-drug use will total $414 billion by 2011, which doesn't include over-the-counter drugs, vitamins, and herbal supplements that can also negatively impact the ecosystem.[3] For example, a natural antidepressant may be beneficial for you but can be toxic to fish, especially when mixed with other chemicals.

According to the Environmental Protection Agency's Website, the PPCPs that are not processed by the human body break down in the environment and enter domestic sewers. Our municipal sewage-treatment plants are not presently engineered specifically for the removal of PPCPs and other unregulated contaminants. The PPCPs also flow into the aquatic environments via sewage, treated sewage sludge (biosolids), and our irrigation systems with reclaimed water. More damage is done as they make their way into the soil.

The Associated Press conducted a five-month investigation and determined that, indeed, pharmaceuticals are moving into the water supply, posing a major threat to biodiversity. These drugs are dangerous to all aquatic species, the environment, and to humans throughout the world. Some fish now have extreme reproductive problems as well as other unusual deformities and health issues.

Author and environmentalist Stephen Buhner notes that Americans ingest 30 billion aspirin each year; after these move through our bodies, they end up in the sewer system. Even though a great deal is removed, large doses can interfere with the ecosystem. He also points out that synthetic pharmaceuticals likely persist rather than break down; and warns that the amount of drugs and agrochemicals produced is enough to disrupt the homeostatic balance of all plant life, ecosystems, and the earth itself. These chemicals can have a magnified impact on the ecosystem in the unpredictable ways in which they interact together and sometimes in the ways they affect plant chemistries. Buhner credits Morris Fishbein, M.D., an editor of the *Journal of the American Medical Association* who died in 1976, as knowing far more than he realized when he stated that modern scientific chemotherapy would "wash away the plant and vegetable debris."[4]

Moreover, Jan Schipper, the director of Global Mammal Assessment at the International Union for the Conservation of Nature, states: "PPCP—this is an emerging field of study, and though I am fairly certain there are some impacts on freshwater and maybe near shore marine species, we are still not certain of the pathways and effects these 'cocktails' will have on mammal fauna."[5] A government official I interviewed, who didn't want to be named, also admitted that "PPCPs have emerged as an issue much faster than the federal government has been able to respond."

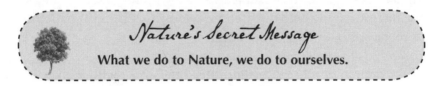

Nature's Secret Message
What we do to Nature, we do to ourselves.

We won't know all the effects until we do more studies. But will it be too late by then? Is it possible that the antibiotics and antimicrobial soaps in the environment are creating "superbugs" (bugs that become resistant to our chemicals and antibiotics)? Could the hormone replacements and birth control pills that have gone into the environment affect the hormones of other species? Could our toxic personal-care and cleaning products be making a mess with the environment? Maybe our best prescription for the health of the planet is to exercise extreme caution in the use of PPCPs and dispose of them safely.

Please review the following information (as well as both appendices) for additional, easy ways to help limit PPCPs. Remember, *you* can help by choosing household and personal-care products that don't contain artificial fragrances, antimicrobials (such as triclosan), BHA (a preservative), or BPA (a chemical contained in some plastics). It's really up to you.

*Summary: Preventing Medicine's Side
Effects on You and the Planet*

Tips to Prevent Mistakes with Your Medications

— Double-check to make sure you have the correct prescription and dosage. Dr. Alen Voskanian, a faculty member at the UCLA School of Medicine, recommends that doctors write prescriptions with a zero prior to the decimal point (0.5) and no zero after (.5) to avoid .500 mg being read as 500 mg; or spell out numbers like on a personal check. In addition, studies have showed that electronic prescribing can catch many dangerous errors.

— Check the side effects, potential drug interactions, and warnings about whether to consume the drug with foods. For example, antibiotics may render birth control pills useless, and grapefruit juice may also dilute a drug's effect.

— Keep in mind that medications can conflict with each other. Let your physician know everything you're taking, including herbs and supplements, and do your own research to discover any potential clashes.

Environmentally Responsible Disposal of Medications

— Do *not* dispose of pharmaceuticals by dumping them down a sink's drain or flushing them in the toilet. (This also applies to vitamins, supplements, and over-the-counter medications.)

— If you throw out unneeded, unused, or expired pharmaceuticals in the trash, "treat" them to prevent exposure to people and animals by adding water, fireplace ashes, or dirt. Or you can take them out of their original containers and secure them in durable packaging before throwing them in the trash.

— If you're a health-care practitioner, instruct your patients on ways to safely and properly dispose of expired and unused prescriptions.

— Check your state's Department of Toxic Substance Control (DTSC) for prescription-drug and toxic-household substance collection sites in your area. California residents can type in their zip code at **www.nodrugsdownthedrain.com** for a list of disposal sites.

— Chemotherapy pharmaceuticals should be returned to the clinic that dispensed them.

— Request that your pharmacy use "green" methods to dispose of medications; **www.greenpharmacyprogram.com** helps communities safely dispose of expired medicines.

"The ability of a bark, leaf, or root to transform the body in a positive manner is a mystery that serves to daily rekindle my passion for the natural world."

— **Darryl Patton, M.A., N.D.**

❦ ❦ ❦   ❦ ❦ ❦

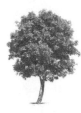

CHAPTER FIFTEEN

Clashing or Harmonizing with Nature?

*"When one tugs at a single thing in nature,
he finds it attached to the rest of the world."*

— **John Muir**

Humans, plants, and animals are all pieces of an intricately magnificent and beautiful puzzle, fitting together just so. If we harm any part of the environment, we'll eventually be harming ourselves. And so when we clash with Nature, we're really sparring with ourselves. We must learn to walk in balance with Mother Nature and take her messages to heart for our health and well-being—and ultimately for our very survival.

In his book *We Talk, You Listen,* published in 1970, Native American advocate Vine Deloria, Jr., argued that pollution, corporate greed, and lack of accountability were destroying the earth:

> Every now and then I am impressed with the thinking of the non-Indian. I was in Cleveland last year and got to talking with a non-Indian about American history. He said that he was really sorry about what happened to Indians, but there was good reason for it. The continent had to be developed and he felt that Indians had stood in the way and thus had had to be removed. "After all,"

he remarked, "what did you do with the land when you had it?" I didn't understand him until later when I discovered that the Cuyahoga River running through Cleveland is inflammable. So many combustible pollutants are dumped into the river that the inhabitants have to take special precautions during the summer to avoid accidentally setting it on fire. After reviewing the argument of my non-Indian friend I decided that he was probably correct. Whites had made better use of the land. How many Indians could have thought of creating an inflammable river?

Repeating the Past?

Are we doing the same things to the inhabitants of the rain forest that we did to the American Indians? Indigenous and tribal peoples are the rightful owners of their land. Their rights should be recognized in law and respected in practice. Nothing should happen on their land without their free, prior, and informed consent. They are the people who know what's best for the rain forest and for themselves.

Today, we think we're smarter and more efficient than tribal cultures and the natural world. We find ways to manipulate Nature and dominate her, not realizing that our disrespect results in our own poor health and increased stress. We're even doing the same thing to insects, using chemicals and changing their natural habitat to fit our wants, oblivious to the dire consequences. Bees are a good example.

"Bee-Leaving"—Are Nature's Messengers Giving Us Profound Warnings?

> "If honeybees became extinct,
> human society would follow in four years."

— **Albert Einstein**

You may have heard about the phenomenon known as Colony Collapse Disorder (CCD), where millions of bees are rapidly vanishing from their hives. So bees are disappearing . . . what's all the fuss about, right? Don't we have more important things to worry about?

Did you know that bees are a $15 *billion* industry? Bee pollination supports about a third of the human diet. If they vanish, then the food you eat that comes from the plants they help pollinate will vanish along with them, never to be seen or tasted again . . . that means almonds, apples, strawberries, blueberries, oranges, peaches, melons, soybeans, cotton, and *more*.

Bees are disappearing worldwide, without a trace. It's unheard of for bees to abandon their hives, and it's downright bizarre that we can't find the missing bodies. Theories abound on the cause of this crisis, including genetically modified pollens; pesticides; poor nutrition; viruses; an unknown fungus; excess stressors; and even the manner in which the hives are abruptly transported from one place to another, disrupting the bees' natural behavioral patterns.

These theories raise more serious questions. Could the bees be sensors for the environment? Are they our "canaries in the coal mine"? Where on earth are they?! Why aren't they returning? (Please see Appendix I for more information on CCD and how you can help our life-giving bees.)

Nature's Secret Message
Generally, animals and insects know what's happening with the planet before we do. Observing them is crucial.

Unnatural Treatment of Animals Could Be Affecting Our Health

> *"And I will send grass in thy fields for thy cattle, that thou mayest eat and be satisfied."*
>
> — **Deuteronomy 11:15**

What needs to be put out to pasture are the ideas that treating animals unnaturally doesn't affect our health. We're interfering with Nature by denying animals free movement and by changing what they typically eat. It's instinctual for them to roam around and graze in pastures; instead, for instance, most dairy cattle are confined in sheds, standing on concrete, deprived of the health benefits of grazing on grass in the fresh air and sunlight.

Likewise, to fatten up beef cattle, we feed them grain in immensely overcrowded areas, which breeds disease. Then we use antibiotics to keep them from getting sick—ignoring the effects that this has on the meat, and in turn, on our health. These unnatural practices also lead to the use of other drugs and irradiation, resulting in even more complications—all because we want Nature on our terms.

Pasture-raised animals receive their vitamins naturally from nutrient-rich, sun-kissed grass. You can counteract the unhealthy trend away from Nature by buying food from only organic free-range animals and fowl that receive their nutrients from living grass, which is rich in vitamin E, vitamin A, beta-carotene, enzymes, and antioxidants that nourish your body. A healthy animal produces healthy food. If you buy dairy products, look for the words *organic* or *grass fed* on the label.

The documentary *Food, Inc.* shows the depressive conditions for both the animals and workers in slaughterhouses. This brutal, inhumane treatment also applies to dolphins, as depicted in the award-winning documentary *The Cove*. If quantum physics is correct and everything is energy, then could the food we eat contain negative energy created by these cruel methods? Could this relate to the fact that the number of people taking antidepressants is increasing at an alarming rate?

And what about the energy of pesticides and other chemicals used? Do you think scrubbing or peeling gets rid of them? Washing helps remove some of them, but how much is absorbed?

Pesticides—More than Meets the Eye

It's often reported that carrots contain high levels of pesticide residue. As an experiment, I put some food coloring on a carrot. When I sliced it, I saw the coloring inside the carrot.

"Hey, wait a minute!" you may say. "You put the food coloring directly on the carrot's skin. When a crop is sprayed with pesticides, they touch only the leaves and soil—not the carrot." This is true, but when I then put food coloring *only* on the carrot's leaves, once again I found dye inside of the carrot.

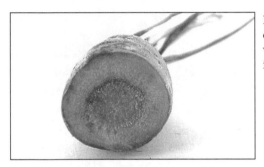

Food coloring was applied only to leaves to test whether pesticides seep into foods.

Naturally, this isn't a scientific experiment, and dye may react differently than pesticides, but the point is that scrubbing and peeling may not remove chemicals entirely. This can explain why carrots are rated high on pesticide levels, even though they are in the ground. Sustain: the alliance for better food and farming states that some pesticides may be systemic, which means they are found inside the carrot and can't be removed by peeling alone, which confirms my experiment. However, the alliance's food facts report that peeling will help remove other pesticides that aren't systemic.

This experiment also shows that separate parts of a plant relate to the entire plant. Raising our perspective one step further, we see that since birds and wildlife feed on carrots, pesticides harm the environment at large. And there are also health risks to farmers associated with these chemicals. One farmer told me that he knew of several farmworkers who had suffered severe side effects from the chemicals that they used, which we now know to be toxic.

On the other hand, organic farmers have figured out many ways to grow healthy food without the use of pesticides and chemicals.

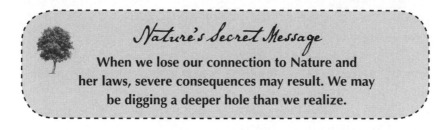

Nature's Secret Message
When we lose our connection to Nature and her laws, severe consequences may result. We may be digging a deeper hole than we realize.

Nature's Cleaners—Powerful and Healthy

A funny thing happened when I was doing the carrot and food-coloring experiment. The dye left a stain on my hands that looked like colored gloves. I thought it would easily come right off . . . wrong! Soap didn't make a bit of difference. Even hydrogen peroxide didn't work. Visions of the Bond girl who died from being painted gold swirled in my head. *Maybe bleach could do the trick,* I thought, *but it's so harsh.* I needed something else. *Hmm.*

As I searched my home for a gentle but effective stain remover, I came across Maggie's Soap Nuts. The slogan on the bag read: "Laundry soap that grows on trees!" I'd received a sample at a health convention but wondered how nuts could clean clothes.

Before I get into that, though, you may be wondering, *What's a "soap nut," anyway?* According to the company's Website, soap nuts are the dried fruit of the Chinese soapberry tree (*Sapindus mukorrosi*), similar to the lychee. Years ago, people in Southeast Asia discovered that when the nuts got wet, they released saponin, a natural cleanser, which made them great for washing clothes. Ancient Indians used them to treat wrinkles and eczema, and soap nuts are also rich in iron and can be eaten to treat anemia. Their rich, deep red color may have been a sign to the ancients that they could benefit blood (as discussed in Chapter 4).

This seemed like a nutty gimmick, but I decided to give them a try. I picked up three soap nuts in my deeply stained hands and added water. Sure enough, the nuts foamed up, and to my surprise, they gently removed the stains. Check out the following photo. Amazing!

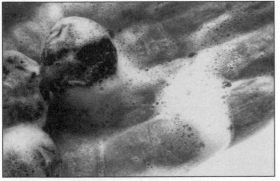

All-natural soap nuts lather with water and gently remove stains.

When I contacted the owner of Maggie's Soap Nuts, Dariel Garner, he explained the dangers of chemical detergents: 60 percent of the rates of infant eczema and 40 percent of child eczema are related to additives in laundry soap. Dariel also told me the story of a friend working in a shampoo factory who truly needs to "suit up" for the job: rubber suit, bubble helmet, and oxygen mask . . . *just to make shampoo!* In contrast, when workers process soap nuts for sale, all they need to don is a hairnet.[1]

Another Way We're Fooling with Nature—GMOs

"Unlabeled GMOs in our food works against what
I have learned in my 30 years as a family farmer.
Agriculture should be sustainable, food should be healthy
and safe, and people deserve to know what they're eating."

— **U.S. senator Jon Tester**

The term "GMO" stands for Genetically Modified Organisms, but my acronym is Gambling with Modified Organisms because numerous health risks have been associated with GMO foods, and the results can be totally unpredictable. A GMO is created when genes from one species have been inserted into another. For example, genes from an Arctic flounder (which can endure cold temperatures) have been spliced into a tomato plant to prevent frost damage. This seems beneficial, yet as Ignacio Chapela, microbial ecologist and mycologist at the University of California, Berkeley, warns: "I think this [genetically modifying foods] is probably the largest biological experiment humanity has ever entered into."[2]

(For more information, the documentary *The Future of Food* offers an in-depth investigation into the disturbing truth behind the unlabeled, patented, genetically engineered foods that have quietly filled U.S. grocery-store shelves for the past decade.)

We've learned how chemically and profoundly complex Nature is, but we still decide to try to "perfect" her and create foods that can last longer on our store shelves. Is shelf life more important than our own lives? What would happen if food companies thought of *self*-life instead?

Many products that contain GMOs aren't labeled. Therefore, look for packages that state: "No GMOs" or "GMO free." You can also look at the stickers on your produce. If the PLU ("price lookup") code starts with the number eight and has five digits total, then it was genetically modified. If the code starts with the number nine, then it was organically grown. And if it's just four digits, it was conventionally grown. Here's a quick breakdown:

- A conventionally grown banana has a four-digit PLU: 4011.

- An organic banana has the number nine at the beginning: 94011. (Remember that nine is fine!)

- A genetically engineered (or genetically modified) banana begins with an eight: 84011.

Unfortunately, labeling cooperation is voluntary and not mandated, and more than 70 percent of our food has been genetically modified. Why can't the sticker just clearly say "organic" or "genetically modified"? Who can keep track of these codes? If we need codes to understand these labels, what about other food labels?

What's Natural in "Natural Flavors"?

Some food labels remind me of résumés—both tend to be embellished! When the words *natural flavors* appear on a label, it may also be giving a glamorized impression. Was this food picked fresh at the farm? According to the Code of Federal Regulations, the definition of the term is a substance "whose significant function in food is flavoring rather than nutritional."

If a label contains "natural flavors," it doesn't mean that it's natural or healthy, as you may have been led to believe. It's not about what it contains. Artificial and natural flavors are manufactured at the same chemical plants, which have nothing to do with Nature. And by the way, the word *organic* on the label means that it's at least 95 percent organic; "100% organic" means just that. Food labels can be so sneaky!

Images and Wording on Food Labels May Be Misleading

Does this symbol mean that the product is healthy?

When I first saw this symbol on my food package, I wasn't sure what it meant. It looked like the sun shining on a plant, earthy and natural, so I assumed it was healthy. I read the words around the logo: "Treated by irradiation for freshness and quality." *I certainly do want fresh, quality food,* I thought.

Let's take a closer look. This "radura" symbol indicates that the food has received high doses of irradiation in the form of electron beams. The FDA claims that this is done to kill harmful insects, parasites, and bacteria, such as E coli; along with inhibiting ripening and sprouting—all without a "significant" difference in the taste or nutrition. However, Wenonah Hauter, executive director of the organization Food & Water Watch, reports differently:

> Scientists have observed serious health problems in lab animals fed irradiated foods. Those include premature death, cancer, tumors, stillbirths, mutations, organ damage, immune system failure and stunted growth. . . . Americans deserve better food safety solutions from their government and the food industry than expensive, impractical, ineffective, and potentially dangerous technologies like irradiation.[3]

The Center for Food Safety, a nonprofit advocacy organization, claims that irradiation produces "a higher cost for low-quality food." The Organic Consumer Association is concerned that the use of irradiation could backfire because food producers may not be taking the necessary steps to ensure the food's safety if they assume that the food will get "cleaned up" with radiation later.

Possible Sources of E Coli, Insects, and Parasites

Doesn't it make more sense to figure out what's *causing* food exposure to the harmful bacteria E coli *before* treating the effects? This reminds me of a fictional story in which a whole town organized rescue teams for injured people found floating downstream in a river. They put all their efforts into medical personnel, ambulances, ways to remove the injured, and building hospitals. Someone finally went upstream only to discover that it was just one individual who was pushing people in the water and causing all the chaos. If the town had first looked for the cause, there would have been no need for all the expense and effort downstream. Likewise, irradiation may be focusing on the wrong issue.

If we check the "upstream" of irradiation, could the overcrowding of animals in an unsanitary environment be the source of the harmful pathogens? Neal Barnard, M.D., nutrition researcher and president of the Physicians Committee for Responsible Medicine, wrote the following in *AgWeek* about consumers being warned to avoid peanut products because of a salmonella outbreak:

> When produce becomes tainted, it's usually because feces from an infected animal contaminated the fertilizer or irrigation water used in the fields. . . . Farm animal waste was the identified cause of the 2006 spinach E. coli outbreak, according to an investigation by the FDA. . . . The original source of this salmonella outbreak is not peanuts—it's our out-of-control factory farming system. . . .
>
> With Georgia's poultry industry raising more than 1.3 billion birds a year in crowded, often unsanitary conditions, it's no surprise that some of the billions of peanuts grown in the state are infected with salmonella and other bacteria. . . . [It's] easy for deadly bacteria to travel through runoff into adjacent fields where peanuts and other crops are grown."[4]

Lack of personal hygiene by workers handling food also causes it to become contaminated. Crop pickers in the fields, without easy access to washrooms, can spread bacteria to the produce. Careless use of plastic gloves is yet another way to spread germs. I remember once at a supermarket, I watched a food demonstrator wearing plastic gloves stop to shake hands, answer his cell phone, use a pen, scratch his head, and then continue handling the food with the same gloves.

In addition, when food is shipped around the world, compromises may have to be made to ensure freshness, often breaking the rules of Nature. Improper food handling is a major factor in E coli, salmonella, and other harmful contamination problems. How are we to know what's being done to our food before we take it home?

"What's in a Name" . . . or Label?

If food is irradiated, it must be labeled as such. But there's a catch: According to an FDA paper on irradiation labeling: "If irradiated ingredients are added to foods that have not been irradiated, no special labeling is required on retail packages." Did you get that? The ingredients added to a product might be irradiated and mum's the word—they don't have to let you know. This labeling also doesn't apply to restaurant or processed foods.

Companies are considering changing *irradiation* to *electronically pasteurized* or *cold pasteurized* to make it sound more appealing. They feel that the word *irradiation* scares people off so they want to alter the labeling on packages. "Cold pasteurized" is so terribly misleading because it sounds like it has taken the heat out to make it better, like our familiar, healthy "cold pressed" oils. I e-mailed a popular meat-service company to inquire if their beef is irradiated. They wrote back using the new term "electronically pasteurized" and explained that it's "ordinary, everyday electricity, which ensures safety against E coli and other dangerous bacteria." *Hmm.*

Even the made-up word *radura* leads to ambiguity, since we have no idea what it means. Why not call it what it is—the irradiation symbol? The organization Sustainable Communities Network comments: "The Radura distracts your attention from the fact that irradiation is mostly about 'sterilizing' food possibly contaminated with feces, not about preserving flowers."

Let's see . . . not labeling all ingredients; using nicer sounding, ambiguous terms; and including an innocent-looking plant logo for irradiation—maybe the words and terms need to get cleaned up so we understand what's actually going on.

Pasteurizing to Save Lives?

Another term that may be misleading is the high-heat process called pasteurizing ("past-your-eyes"). Have you ever wondered why fresh-squeezed orange juice tastes so much better than the juice you buy at the store? Most store-bought juices are pasteurized, which means they're heated at high temperatures, which kills not only bacteria but also some valuable nutrients and enzymes. Pasteurization affects the flavor and integrity of the juice. "Flash pasteurization" is somewhat less destructive, since the juice is heated for a shorter period of time, then cooled to retain more nutrients.

Because of the nutritional damage that pasteurization inflicts, some juice companies want to offer unpasteurized juice to consumers, but the FDA won't permit it.

Would You Drink Unpasteurized Milk?

You may be thinking, *Omigawd, unpasteurized milk! That's so unsafe!* Before you put this idea out to pasture, take a moment to consider the facts: in more than 32 million servings of unpasteurized milk from the company Organic Pastures (offered in California), and after more than five years of intensive testing (more testing than past-your-eyes milk), not one single pathogen was detected. Did you get that? Not a single pathogen.

Mark McAfee, the president of Organic Pastures, asserts that his raw organic milk is tested 50 times more strictly than pasteurized milk:

> Our cows have no antibiotics or hormones used, and are fed so well they don't even have pathogens. This change in physiology directly inhibits pathogen development in the milk (a transfer from environmental contamination doesn't seem to occur; there are no 'bad bugs' in the manure that transfer into the milk, and the clean raw milk is highly pathogen resistant). So clean, pure cows equal clean pure milk. We feel that if there is suffering of the cow, there is suffering of the milk.[5]

Happy, healthy cows make healthy milk. One action affects another action.

Nature's Web—Everything Is Connected

Scientists laughed at the Navajo Indians' protests: "If you kill off the prairie dogs, there will be no one to cry for the rain." It made no sense. They didn't see any relevance or connections. In the 1950s, all the prairie dogs in the area around Chilchinbito, Arizona, were killed because people thought it would protect the desert grasses. That area became a desolate wasteland.

Stephen Buhner, in his book *One Spirit Many Peoples,* explains what went wrong:

> Prairie dogs and all the burrowing creatures open breathing tubes in the Earth. As the moon circles the Earth, it pulls on the underground aquifers, just as it pulls on the oceans to cause the tides. This pull on the underground aquifers, causing them to rise and fall, is akin to the breathing process in human bodies. As the underground waters rise and fall, the Earth literally breathes through the fissures created by the burrowing creatures. The Earth breathes out moisture-laden air, which helps to create rain.[6]

Various types of wildlife can hang out in the prairie dogs' burrows—but not after the prairie dogs were killed. The Navajo Indians knew the importance of how one animal is part of, and contributes to, the whole of the system. The interdependency between mammals, fungi, organisms, and even invisible microbes is very complex. And it's not only animals that are interconnected—it's all of Nature, just like the popular concept of "six degrees of separation." Generally, if you change one thing in Nature, it eventually affects everything else.

Nature's Secret Message
**All of Nature is interconnected,
including the human race.**

Mind, Body, Soul . . . and the Environment

We've all heard of the mind-body connection. Then *spirit* or *soul* was added to show that there was another piece to the equation. However, we also need to include the environment. We don't operate in a bubble. Our surroundings, which include Nature and other people, too, are the intricate connections that dramatically affect our mind, body, and soul.

We're like the prairie dogs, in the sense that if you remove one part in the food-supply chain, it will affect the whole. For instance, think of all the people involved in order for you to buy food whenever you need it. There are those who gather and sell the seeds, farmers, water-supply companies, harvesters, truckers, store buyers, accountants, and grocery-store personnel—and that's not even mentioning the individuals who produce the trucks to transport the food, manufacture the bags to hold the food, and so on. Just like the prairie dogs, if you remove one part (or person), it affects the whole system.

I recall playing in the garden in the springtime when I was a kid. I kept running across big ol' gooey, slimy, slippery worms; and I'd let out a squeal. *Eeeew!* From my perspective, they were ruining my mom's garden! Then my mom told me how they aerate the soil, creating healthy food. They were a garden's greatest helpers. These worms were actually "change agents," helping the soil transition. It was my first glimpse into understanding how various elements of Nature, working together as a whole, were part of a grand design beyond my limited comprehension.

When scientists extract one compound from a plant or food, it lacks the other nutrients needed to function as a whole. Mother Nature has knit everything together for the good of all. The Internet (or World Wide Web) is a great metaphor for how everything is connected in Nature.

One action affects another. Farmers growing organic avocados told me that they want an ordinance for the nonorganic farmers to not be able to spray pesticides when it's windy since the chemicals blow onto their crops. Our pesticides don't only kill pests, but they also have an effect on the food, soil, future food, rivers, farmers, and wildlife. We can no longer afford to ignore how we've dominated and mistreated Mother Nature and that the toxins we've put in the environment are now negatively affecting us. So why do we care? Because when we look into Nature's eyes, we see our own.

Cheap food mirrors our charge-card economy. We want it now, but we don't think to look at how we may pay in compounded interest in practically all areas of our lives down the line.

Shop the Vote!

MTV has a huge campaign called "Rock the Vote," which is designed to help young people get registered to vote and interested in the political system. But it's also important to "shop the vote," meaning that what you buy is a vote for that food or product. The dollars you spend cast your vote and can make a huge impact on business. For example, Walmart now sells organic items because there was a demand for it. If no one buys a product, that product will go out of business. What you buy and don't buy makes a powerful statement to business and government.

Next time you're comparing prices, consider the overall costs to your health, the environment, the health-care system, and the planet. Nonorganic products may be cheaper, but they're actually more costly in the long run because the pesticides they contain have been linked to cancer, obesity, Alzheimer's, and some birth defects, which create huge medical bills.

Second, it's adversely affecting rivers, soil, oceans, wildlife, farmers, and consumers. It's scientifically proven that healthy food creates healthy people. Taking care of your health means less heath care is needed, and that brings the price of health care down.

Valuable nutrients are removed in processed food, which is cheap, but costly to your health in the long run. Money saved can be a bypass earned.

> ### *Nature's Secret Message*
> **When we harm Nature, we harm ourselves.**

We're now in a world where we can no longer just look at prices—we need to look at the costs involved in buying each food or product. As Martin Luther King, Jr., stated: "Whatever affects one directly, affects all indirectly. . . . This is the interrelated structure of reality."

If something comes from a company that mistreats its workers or from a corporation that rapes the land or inhumanely treats animals, then that cheap product is very expensive to both you and society. When you're shopping, ask yourself, *What's the cost of pollution to the land and the damage to the soil? What's the cost of the negative energy and cruelty to the animals and workers? How much fuel does it take to ship a fruit from around the world so I can have it out of season? What's done to the food to "clean it up"?*

There's so much you can do to help. (Many simple steps are listed in the appendices at the end of the book.) The following, written on the tomb of an 11th-century Anglican bishop at Westminster Abbey, sums up the power you have in your individual actions:

> *When I was young and free and my imagination had no limits, I dreamed of changing the world. As I grew older and wiser, I discovered the world would not change, so I shortened my sights somewhat and decided to change only my country.*
>
> *But it, too, seemed immovable.*
>
> *As I grew into my twilight years, in one last desperate attempt, I settled for changing only my family, those closest to me, but alas, they would have none of it.*
>
> *And now as I lie on my deathbed, I suddenly realized: If I had only changed myself first, then by example I would have changed my family.*
>
> *From their inspiration and encouragement, I would then have been able to better my country, and who knows, I may have even changed the world.*

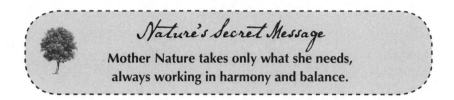

Nature's Secret Message

**Mother Nature takes only what she needs,
always working in harmony and balance.**

Nature gives us harmony and balance. Native Americans believe in giving back to the land. A medicine man respectfully asks permission from the plant to harvest it and then offers prayers of gratitude for the plant's blessings and energies bestowed on them. The entire plant is used, and part of the root is planted back in the soil so it can regenerate.

Nature mirrors us and shows us we're all connected, so we must remember that whatever we do to Nature, we do to ourselves. As we discussed earlier, it's obvious that there's a connection between the fact that the most commonly prescribed drugs in America are antidepressants and that we spend less time in Nature than ever before. Mother Nature's prescription of connecting with something divine is right there for us.

An instant relaxer and antidepressant for anyone is to go to a natural setting, sit on the ground, and feel the earth's support and energy of the trees. Have you ever seen a vacation ad that says "Stay inside all day!" No! Instead, brochures are filled with scenes of azure seas and white beaches or skiing or hiking in majestic mountains, all beckoning with the promise of recreation and renewal.

This connection and respect for Nature is vital today for the health and well-being of society. Are you willing to take steps to give back to the earth to complete the circle? Mother Nature is there for you. Are you there for her?

> *"When you know nature as part of yourself,
> you will act in harmony. When you feel yourself part
> of nature, you will live in harmony."*
>
> — Tao Te Ching

232

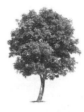

AFTERWORD

*"There are only two ways to live your life: One is
as though nothing is a miracle. The other is as though
everything is a miracle. I believe in the latter."*

— Albert Einstein

Today while walking in Nature, I noticed star-shaped, closed buds that looked like buttons. As I stopped to marvel, a lizard climbed up the tree and stopped right in front of me, two feet from my face. There we were, eye to eye. Time stood still. I couldn't remember the last time I saw a lizard, or maybe I just never noticed one before.

I'd read about how lizards shed their skin—a symbol for letting go of the old and making way for new beginnings. A lizard can also break off its tail to distract a predator in order to escape and then later regrow it. Even our smartest researchers haven't figured out how we can regrow a limb—something that the lizard does naturally!

I suddenly saw the symbolism in my life as I was finishing the very last pages of this book. As I said good-bye to the lizard, my ancient-looking friend, I realized it was time to say good-bye to old ways, finish the book, and welcome what new journey awaits. To me, that's a secret of being at one with Nature. She sparks creativity and imagination, whether symbolically or literally, so that we can see, think, and feel in new ways.

I've heard of herb classes in which the first exercise is to find your favorite plant, or a plant that "calls to you." Wouldn't you know it that most times, the plant that students choose is the one that has the correct remedy specifically for them! And I just read about the Moringa tree and that all of its parts (the bark, seed-pods, flowers, leaves, and roots) are not only edible but also vastly nutritious—far more so than corn, wheat, and soy. The Moringa's seed-kernel powder can even be used to purify water. Imagine that—all that genius in one species of tree! Just think what other healing secrets are yet to be discovered in Nature's bounty.

However, there's far more to our relationship with Nature than figuring out how many ways we can benefit from its beauty and wisdom. When we discover the joy in our connectedness with Mother Nature, we will long to nurture her. We must be mindful to follow the universal law of balancing what we take with what we give.

Even being willing to take small, simple steps to care for the environment (like those listed in the appendices, for example) can go a long way toward restoring that balance. Hopefully, the more you look for and learn about Nature's infinite wisdom, the more she will reveal her secrets—and the more you'll learn how to express your gratitude and love for this precious planet.

After all, Mother Nature, your friend and mentor, is always there for you. She's willing to guide you in every step you take. To hear her whispers and absorb her secrets is so easy to do . . . simply stop, look, and listen.

🍃 🍃 🍃   🍃 🍃 🍃

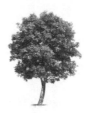

Simple Ways You Can Save Money and the Planet

"Never doubt that a small group of thoughtful committed citizens can change the world; indeed, it's the only thing that ever has."

— **Margaret Mead**

I have the following links and more links, information, and secrets on my Website: **www.ElaineWilkes.com**.

Bees—Colony Collapse Disorder

— Are you a "bee-liever" that there may be a dire message coming from these extraordinary little creatures? Why not increase native honeybee populations by planting bee-friendly plants in your yard, or anywhere outside? Flowers and plants that will attract the attention of bees and humans alike include lavender, glory bushes, jasmine, rosemary, coreopsis, violets, thyme, bluebells, trumpet vine, wisteria, cosmos, coneflowers, and sunflowers. Bees love these plants.

— To find out more on this issue, you might want to take your honey to the thought-provoking documentary *The Vanishing of the Bees* (**http://vanishingbees.com**). You may be inspired to send your friends bee-mails so swarms of people can act on this shocking situation.

— Visit: **www.helpthehoneybees.com**.

— Avoid using pesticides.

— Donate to the Honeybee Research Fund at Penn State and UC Davis, who are conducting studies to help combat Colony Collapse Disorder:

- Penn State: **https://secure.ddar.psu.edu/GiveTo/**

- UC Davis: **https://awc.ucdavis.edu/makeagift .aspx?alloccat=2000**

— We need to be like worker bees to create a big buzz about solving this crisis. To request more funding for this urgent issue, write to:

> Hon. Dennis Cardoza
> House Committee on Agriculture, Subcommittee
> on Horticulture and Organic Agriculture
> 435 Cannon Building
> Washington, DC 20515

Cell-Phone Recycling

Recycle your old cell phones. Cell Phones for Soldiers is a terrific nonprofit organization that provides donated phones to soldiers who are overseas so they can keep in touch with family members. Visit: **www.cellphonesforsoldiers.com** to find a drop-off location or to print a prepaid shipping label.

Cleaning Green

— Did you know that it's suspected that stay-at-home moms get more diseases because they're breathing in toxic cleaning chemicals? You can make your own cleaners that will save money, your health, and the environment. Reuse your spray bottles, and fill them with the following:

- *All-purpose cleaner:* You can use this on hard surfaces such as countertops and kitchen floors, as well as windows and mirrors. Mix equal parts of white distilled vinegar and water. Add a few drops of essential oil for fragrance, if desired.

- *Toilet-bowl cleaner:* Mix baking soda (get non-aluminum at health-food stores) and vinegar. Watch it fizz up, then scrub away.

— Many commercial dry cleaners offer to clean clothes using nontoxic chemicals. Ask to go plastic free or have all of your clothes wrapped in one plastic bag.

Cosmetics

What's in your makeup and beauty products? Did you know that the FDA doesn't require companies to test the safety of cosmetic products before manufacturing? Be sure to buy eco-friendly products that contain no toxic ingredients. The Campaign for Safe Cosmetics provides a wealth of articles and information as well as a terrific database to look up the ingredients in your personal-care products: **www.safecosmetics.org**.

Creating Communities That
Support People and the Planet

— Have you ever heard of a "conservation community"? Prairie Crossing is a critically acclaimed community in Illinois that was designed to combine responsible development, the preservation of open land, and easy commuting by rail. Find out more on their Website: **www.prairiecrossing.com**.

— Check with your city regarding plots they inexpensively "rent" out for gardening. You can Google the words *garden plot* with your town's name in the search box. Most incorporated cities have garden-plot rentals.

Earth Hour—You Turn Me Off

The World Wildlife Fund is asking individuals, businesses, governments, and organizations around the world to turn off their lights for one hour—Earth Hour—to make a global statement of concern about climate change and to demonstrate a commitment to finding solutions. For more information, visit: **www.EarthHourUS.org** and **www.EarthHourKids.org**.

Eco-Disposal

— Prevent pharmaceutical pollution! Visit **www.greenpharmacy program.com**.

— Ask your health-care provider to inform patients about proper drug disposal.

— Dispose of CFL lightbulbs responsibly or recycle them. Don't throw them in the trash! For more info, go to: **www.epa.gov/bulb recycling**. Or bring them to ACE Hardware or Home Depot.

— Bring your batteries to stores such as RadioShack and Whole Foods Market, and they'll properly dispose of them for you.

— Not sure how to dispose of paper, metal, hazardous, plastic, glass, electronics, automotive, household, garden, and construction waste? The Website **http://earth911.com** tells all.

Electricity Conservation

— Even if things are plugged in and turned off, they still suck energy and use about 10 percent of your electric bill! So unplug when not in use.

— Why not save money on electricity by turning lights, TVs, and radios off when not needed? Ask your company to cut down on their electricity usage at night while no one is there.

— Become energy conscious while traveling, too! When you're staying at a motel, it's so simple to turn everything off when you leave the room. Some hotels even have one turn-off switch for all the lights in the room, which is a great idea.

Farmers' Market

Support local farmers! You'll get healthier, tastier, and in many cases, less expensive food. Visiting your neighborhood's farmers' market is also a great way to stay connected with your community.

Footprint—What's Your Global Impact?

Check out the Personal Footprint calculator (**www.footprint network.org**), and find out how much you're helping or hurting global warming.

Forests—Conserving and Protecting

Studies show that ADD and stress are reduced when in Nature, so visit a national park or forest. National-park visitation is down 55 percent. Visit the following Websites:

- **http://theloraxproject.com/**
- **www.nps.gov**

Gardening

You can start organic gardening right away with this all-in-one kit: **www.Minifarmbox.com.**

Global Warming

Laurie David (the producer of *An Inconvenient Truth*), Robert F. Kennedy, Jr., and Senator John McCain founded the Stop Global Warming Virtual March to inform people about climate change and combat global warming.

For cool ideas to save the planet and money, check out their excellent "Take Action Tips" at: **www.stopglobalwarming.org/sgw_actionitems.asp.**

Insecticides and Pest Control

— Use organic botanical products instead of chemicals. Check out EcoSmart at: **http://ecosmart.com.**

— Instead of using toxic bug killers for household plants, make a mixture of dish soap and water, spray it on the plants, and rinse. This does the trick for pennies without those toxic chemicals. Or you can also use nontoxic, ready-made pest-control products: **www.allnaturalpestcontrol.net.**

Laundry

Always use cold water. In addition, try substituting a half cup of baking soda (aluminum free) to cut down on the amount of detergent per load. You don't need all that soap! The machine's agitation helps clean the clothes.

For more tips, look up "Laundry Room" in the Home & Garden section on the Green Guide: **www.thegreenguide.com.**

Paper

Here are a couple of tips on recycling paper products and reducing your use:

- Shred your documents and use them as packing material in boxes.

- Use old T-shirts for rags rather than paper towels.

Pets

You can donate used rugs, towels, sheets, blankets, and other bedding to your local animal shelter or veterinarian. They can use these to pad cages, dry animals after baths, and clean up messes.

Plant a Tree

Go outside and plant a tree! Did you know that a single tree will absorb one ton of carbon dioxide? A single California avocado tree can absorb as much carbon dioxide as is produced by a car driven 26,000 miles! In addition, turn off electronic devices. Simply turning off your television, DVD player, stereo, and computer when you're not using them will save thousands of pounds of carbon dioxide each year.

Plastic—BYOB (Bring Your Own Bag)

— Where do plastic bags end up? Understand how the use of plastic bags hurts marine life and the environment. Watch this powerful slideshow: **www.poconorecord.com/apps/pbcs.dll/ article?AID=/20080506/MULTIMEDIA02/80505016.**

— Bring reusable bags with you wherever you shop, or put small purchases in your pockets or purse. When you shop, make it your motto to say, "I have my own bags, thank you."

Recycling

— *Question:* How many plastic bottles are purchased in the United States every year? *Answer:* 90 billion. That's 90,000,000,000 plastics each year! Not only do these bottles require massive amounts of fossil fuel to manufacture and transport (and will eventually fill up landfills), but they also cause havoc in our ecosystem and health. Many plastics contain BPA (bisphenol A) and PVCs (polyvinyl chloride), which are xenoestrogens that can leach into bottles. Visit The Good Human for more info: **http://www.thegoodhuman .com/2008/03/17/choosing-a-safe-reusable-water-bottle/**.

— Why buy water in plastic bottles in the first place? You can purchase a water filter and fill up in glass or steel containers at home. Two million plastic beverage bottles are used in the U.S. every five minutes.

— Recycle at your workplace. Why not bring bottles home to recycle? Or request that your employers start recycling and buying office products that contain recycled material.

— Ever wonder what to recycle? Check the code on the bottom: the numbers 1 through 5 can be recycled, but you need to bring a number 7 to a recycling center. Find out what you can toss in your recycle bin for curbside pickup. (You may be able to conveniently recycle more things than you realize.) Check out: **www .co.hunterdon.nj.us/depts/parks/virtualtours/arb/pic16.htm**.

— Earth 911 contains a wealth of information and articles on recycling. Visit: **http://earth911.com**.

Schools: Remember the Three R's—
Reduce, Reuse, Recycle

— Reuse papers sent home with students (and then recycle them). To save paper and time, ask teachers to e-mail notices to parents.

— Encourage your children to use both sides of paper for assignments.

— According to **Lunchopolis.com:** "On average, every American school-age child throws out 67 pounds of juice boxes, water bottles, aluminum foil and plastic sandwich bags per year. With 25 million children carrying lunch to school daily, that means 3.5 billion pounds of lunchbox garbage are created in America every year."

- **lunchopolis.com** (lead-free, insulated lunch boxes)

- **www.laptoplunches.com** (American-style bento boxes)

- **www.wrap-n-mat.com** (reusable sandwich/
  snack-food wraps)

— Start a gardening program (whether in pots or on a plot of land) for students to learn firsthand about growing vegetables. To see how this has been done, check out: **www.thelearninggarden.org/aboutus.html**.

- **www.edibleschoolyard.org** (instructions for starting a school garden for kids and grown-ups alike)

— What about assigning "light monitors"? Each child at school takes turns switching off lights in empty rooms. It will save the school system a lot of money and teach children the habit of conserving energy.

Shipping

Use your office paper that has been shredded for packing boxes. Save packing popcorn to reuse when you ship.

Water—Saving Our Precious Resource

According to the organization Food & Water Watch, one out of every six people doesn't have access to clean drinking water. Try these conservation tips:

- Ask restaurants owners not to provide glasses of water unless requested.

- Do you really need to let the water run while you brush your teeth? Pick up an inexpensive Smart Faucet for your sinks to eliminate water waste, saving 15,000 gallons per year: **www.water-saver-faucet.com**.

- Fix a leaky faucet and save 20 gallons of water a day or 140 gallons a week.

- Use a broom to clean sidewalks and driveways instead of a hose, and save 150 gallons.

- Save 25 gallons simply by watering your yard before 8 A.M. to reduce evaporation.

- If you have a reverse-osmosis water filter, collect the extra water and use it for watering plants instead of having the extra water run wastefully down the drain.

- Put a bucket in your shower to catch water while it's heating up. Use it for plants or to clean patios.

- Run the water in your faucet the size of a pencil wide. No need to blast it on.

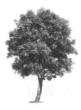

APPENDIX II

Recommended Links and Products

"It is time to make peace with the planet."

— Al Gore

While researching the material for this book, I came upon products and information that I found to be valuable. You can find many more references and products that I've carefully selected on my Website: **www.ElaineWilkes.com**. Here are some of my favorites:

Ayurveda

Dr. Vasant Lad is an author and a world-renown expert on Ayurveda. He gives lectures throughout the country and advice on which herbs to use: **www.friendsofayurveda.com**.

Barbecuing—All-Natural Charcoal Briquettes

Try out these natural charcoal briquettes. They're a carbon-neutral product and are made from trees subject to strict forest-management techniques that naturally regrow after they're harvested: **www.greenheartsbriquette.com**.

Bath Salts

Holistic Skin Food sells mustard bath salts and numerous non-toxic skin-care products: **http://holisticskinfood.com**.

Cleansing and Juice Fasting

iZOCleanze produces raw, vegan, organic juices and superfood cleanses: **www.izocleanze.com**.

Color Therapy

Leslie Sloane is an expert color therapist and the founder and developer of Auracle's Colour Therapy. She conducts workshops and is also available for phone consultations: **www.auraclescolour.com**.

Composting

Tom Szaky, CEO of organic fertilizer company Terracycle, gives reasons why you may wish to compost: "Making compost reduces trash, creates free soil fertilizer, helps soil to retain moisture and resist erosion, improves garden yields, turns waste into a valuable resource, saves limited landfill space, and recycles nutrients back into the soil."

You can compost even if you live in an apartment. Check out: **http://life.gaiam.com/gaiam/p/Why-Compost.html** for several instructional videos to get you started and composting alternatives that make it easy, bug free, and clean.

Crock-Pots—Quick, Healthy, Inexpensive Meals

Feel like you have no time to make meals? It takes just minutes to put ingredients into a Crock-Pot before bedtime or before going to work. You can prepare oatmeal, soups, rice and beans, and so much more. In the morning, or when arriving home from work, you'll have a warm, inexpensive, nourishing meal waiting for you.

Dehydrators

Drying your own food makes nutritious on-the-go snacks, and it's easy to do. You'll save money, especially when you buy food in bulk or dehydrate leftovers. Think of how you'll be helping Mother Nature since you won't be using all that packaging. Here are a few points to consider when buying a dehydrator:

1. Make sure it has a thermostat so you can keep the temperature below 118 degrees to preserve enzymes.

2. A timer will save money and energy.

3. You can purchase nonstick sheets called Paraflexx for easy, stick-free cleanup.

I recommend the brand Good4U because it's quieter and less expensive than other models, and it has a ten-year warranty. It's sold at **www.vitalityplus1.com**—they'll price match.

The ancients would sun dry their foods. (There's Nature at work again!) Now there are solar-powered dehydrators, which you can buy or even make yourself. Google "solar-powered dehydrators" for instructions.

Fibonacci Information

- Gary Meisner, "The Phi Guy": **www.goldennumber.net**

- Jill Britton: **http://britton.disted.camosun.bc.ca/fibslide/jbfibslide.htm**

Films on Food and Environmentalism

- *The Cove* is an engrossing and heartfelt documentary about the slaughtering of dolphins in Japan, which has won numerous awards including Audience Award at the Sundance Film Festival: **http://thecovemovie.com**.

- *Food, Inc.* is terrific! It shows what really goes on in producing our food. Large companies ignore Nature's laws and our health in order to gain profit: **http://robert kennerfilms.com**.

- *The Future of Food* is a documentary about GMO foods. It's a must-see! Go to: **www.thefutureoffood.com**.

- *Generation Rx* is a film about overprescribing children with drugs. I've just seen the trailer—even that was informative: **www.generationrxfilm.com**.

- *The Vanishing of the Bees* is a documentary on Colony Collapse Disorder: **www.vanishingbees.com**.

- *In Good Heart: Soil and the Mystery of Fertility* is by the same director of *The Future of Food*. It examines what we're doing to the soil around the world and how it will affect us: **www.ingoodheart.com**.

- *Fresh* is a new way of thinking about what we're eating: **www.freshthemovie.com**.

- *Simply Raw* is a documentary about diabetics who were able to stop taking their medications after eating a healthy diet for 30 days: **www.rawfor30days.com**.

Flower-Essence Experts

- If you question if flower essences work, check out the before and after photos on this Website: **www.floralive.com/ stories-floralive-flower-essences.htm.**

- David Dalton, founder and director of Delta Gardens Flower Essences: **www.deltagardens.com**

- Joanne Cohen: **www.sacredpassageways.com**

GMO Food Facts

- **www.thefutureoffood.com**
- **www.centerforfoodsafety.org**
- **www.SeedsOfDeception.com**
- **www.seedalliance.org**
- **www.saynotogmos.org**

Herbalist

- Matthew Wood: **www.matthewwoodherbs.com/ Mattwood.html**

Irradiation Information

- **www.organicconsumers.org/irrad/irradfact.cfm**
- **www.sustainabletable.org**
- **www.foodandwaterwatch.org**

Juicers

I have a Green Star juicer, priced around $439. It seems like a lot of money, but I found that I saved money on produce because it extracts more juice (resulting in dry pulp), which means I get the most value from my fruits and vegetables. The slower action retains important enzymes and nutrients, although it takes much longer to juice.

I also have a less expensive juicer, Jack LaLanne's Power Juicer, which costs around $100. I especially like the large feed chute because it saves a lot of cutting time. However, it's loud and creates heat, which destroys enzymes, but it takes less time to use.

What do you do with the leftover pulp? You can put it in a large pot of water and simmer it on the stove for an hour or two, or put it in a Crock-Pot on low. Strain and enjoy a tasty broth that you can eat plain or use as a soup stock for cooking. You can also put a bit back into your drink or compost the pulp.

If you don't have a juicer, you can combine a variety of greens (such as celery, kale, and parsley) with an apple and a peeled, whole lemon in a blender for a quick energy-boosting soup.

Junk Mail

MailStopper will reduce your junk mail by 90 percent, and will plant five trees and monitor your mail for $20 a year: **http:// mailstopper.tonic.com**.

Lice (Nontoxic Removal)

Topanga Alchemy sells a natural, nontoxic formula that's guaranteed to remove head lice. They also carry an all-natural mosquito repellent and products for pets: **www.topangaalchemy.com**.

Mud (Therapeutic Treatments and Facials)

Both of these women can ship their mud-therapy products anywhere in the U.S.:

- Vicki Nevarde (also known as "The Mud Queen"): 619-417-1800

- Lisa Klinker: 858-699-8444

Noise Suppressors for Hydraulic Equipment

The company Wilkes & McLean carries suppressors that are guaranteed to greatly reduce noise and stop shock and pulsation damage to equipment, as well as boosting employees' hearing and morale from not working in such dreadfully noisy environments: **www.WilkesandMcLean.com**.

Ovens

The NuWave Oven is a small, infrared counter oven that saves up to 85 percent of the energy of a conventional oven. It pays for itself in about seven months: **www.nuwaveoven.com**.

Permaculture

The Permaculture Institute (**www.permaculture.org**) will open the door to this fascinating agricultural system.

Pesticide Watch

- PesticideWise is an interactive Website created by the University of California at Riverside that allows you to find critical information on almost any pesticide: **www.pw.ucr.edu**.

- The Pesticide Action Network of North America (PANNA), a nonprofit organization that promotes alternatives to pesticides, includes profiles of orange and apple farmers who made the switch from conventional production to pesticide-free production: **www.panna.org**.

- The Northwest Coalition for Alternatives to Pesticides protects people and the environment by advancing healthy solutions to pest problems: **www.pesticide.org**.

Playgrounds

Play-Well uses shredded tires as a nontoxic ground cover for playgrounds that looks like bark but is bouncy and soft, making the ground safe for kids. Combine two different colors so it looks like mulch: **www.play-well.com/07_our_childrens_future.html**.

Prescription Medicines

- Print out the "Ten Rules for Safer Drug Use" before seeing your doctor: **www.worstpills.org**.

- Lists of drugs for help with patients over 65 are available at: **www.tahsa.org/files%2FDDF%2Fmedbeer1.pdf**.

Pump It Up

No time to juice every day? Why not juice large batches of produce at one time? Freshly squeezed, refrigerated juice can last about four days if you store it in an 8-ounce Ball jar and remove any air by pumping it out. (I got my pump from **www.vitalityplus1 .com**.) Studies show that your body can process only 8 ounces of juice per hour, so storing the juice in 8-ounce jars is ideal.

Raw Food

- Essential Living Foods offers high-quality superfoods, nuts, raw cacao, olives, and more. The company practices conscious business, in which small farmers are supported with sustainable farming techniques: **www.essentialliving foods.com**.

- Famous chef Juliano makes the tastiest raw food on the planet. The Website sells raw food, "uncook" books, and equipment: **www.planetraw.net**.

Reclaimed Building Materials

According to their Website (**http://freegreenexchange .com**): "Free Green Exchange is a free site that allows contractors to post surplus materials that would otherwise be wasted or disposed of at their cost. These needed materials would be picked up or delivered to someone in need of them for little to no money. The reclaimed material is kept out of the landfills and helps create a sustainable world."

Skin Care

You don't have to use harsh chemicals to help your skin. I use and really like the Dermasonic skin-care brush with ultrasonic vibrations. It rejuvenates the skin in a natural manner: **www .HealthToYourDoor.com**.

Sunblock

For Nontoxic sunblock (and other all-natural products), visit: **www.keys-soap.com**.

Wilderness Adventures on the West Coast

www.StevenKHarper.com

Wild-Food Lectures on the East Coast

"Wildman" Steve Brill teaches courses on edible and medicinal wild plants, Nature, and ecology: **www.wildmanstevebrill.com**.

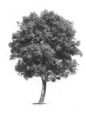

ENDNOTES

Chapter One

[1]Wood, M., phone interview, October 23, 2008.

[2]Weingarten, G., "Pearls Before Breakfast," *The Washington Post,* April 8, 2007: W10.

[3]Eamon, W., *Science and the Secrets of Nature: Books of Secrets in Medieval and Early Modern Culture.* Princeton, NJ: Princeton University Press, 1994.

Chapter Two

[1]Somers, S., *Breakthrough: Eight Steps to Wellness.* New York: Crown Publishers, 2008.

[2]Blue, K., personal communication, September 23, 2008.

[3]California Walnut Board, "Nutrition & Health," **www.walnuts.org/ health/index.php**.

[4]Larsen, J., "Vitamin A & Carotenes," **www.dietitian.com**.

[5]NutritionData, "Know What You Eat," **www.nutritiondata.com**.

[6]Rose, D., phone interview, February 28, 2009.

[7]Murad, H., e-mail correspondence, March 6, 2009.

[8]Heber, D., and S. Bowerman, *What Color Is Your Diet? The 7 Colors of Health.* New York: Regan Books, 2001.

[9]Lutein Information Bureau, "Lutein and Women's Health," **www .luteininfo.com/women**.

[10]Miles, B., phone interview, August 15, 2008.

[11]Etheridge, G., personal interview, September 23, 2008.

[12]POM, "Health Benefits," **www.pomwonderful.com/health_benefits .html**.

[13]Kreitzer, L., phone interview, August, 26, 2008.

[14]Pitchford, P., *Healing with Whole Foods: Asian Traditions and Modern Nutrition.* 3rd ed. Berkeley, CA: North Atlantic Books, 2002.

[15]Seitz, J., e-mail correspondence, May 12, 2009.

Chapter Three

[1]Duke, J.A., with M.J. Bogenschutz-Godwin and A.R. Ottesen, *Duke's Handbook of Medicinal Plants of Latin America.* Boca Raton, FL: Taylor & Francis, 2009.

[2]Taylor, L., *Herbal Secrets of the Rainforest: The Healing Power of Over 50 Medicinal Plants You Should Know About.* Rocklin, CA: Prima Pub., 1998.

[3]Lans, C., "Ethnomedicines Used in Trinidad and Tobago for Reproductive Problems," *Journal of Ethnobiology and Ethnomedicine,* vol. 3, no. 13, 2007.

[4]King, F., and R. Steiner, *Rudolf Steiner and Holistic Medicine.* York Beach, ME: Nicolas-Hays: 1987.

[5]Dalton, D., personal interview, February 16, 2009: **www.deltagardens.com.**

[6]Worley, L., e-mail correspondence, March 18, 2009.

[7]Meissner, M., e-mail correspondence, April 18, 2009.

Chapter Four

[1]Bennett, B., personal interview, August, 8, 2007.

[2]Pichersky, E., and N. Dudareva, "Scent Engineering: Toward the Goal of Controlling How Flowers Smell," *Trends in Biotechnology,* 2007: **www.mcdb.lsa.umich.edu/labs/pichersky/references/Scentengineering.pdf.**

[3]Jubb, D., personal interview, April 29, 2009.

[4]Meadows, R., "Ship Noise Stresses Freshwater Fish," *Conservation* magazine, April–June 2006.

[5]Stiteler, S., e-mail correspondence, October 23, 2008.

[6]Chu, Y., "An Apple a Day May Keep the Doctor Away," *New Scientist,* March 26, 2005.

[7]Robertson, G.S., phone interview, March 11, 2009.

[8]Rupasinghe, V., phone interview, February 11, 2009.

[9]Heber, D., and S. Bowerman, *What Color Is Your Diet? The 7 Colors of Health.* New York: Regan Books, 2001.

[10]Gross, P., "Anthocyanin Antioxidants—Just the Facts," **www.berrywiseinc.com.**

[11]Amber, R.B., *Color Therapy: Healing with Color.* Santa Fe, NM: Aurora Press, 1983.

[12]Sloane, L., personal interview, July 12, 2008.

[13]Dyer, W., "Here's How I Write," **www.drwaynedyer.com/blog/latest.**

[14]Buhner, S.H., *The Lost Language of Plants: The Ecological Importance of Plant Medicines to Life on Earth.* White River Junction, VT: Chelsea Green, 2002.

Chapter Five

[1]Casey, T., personal interview and e-mail, April 14, 2009.

[2]Easterling, J., "Amazon John Easterling & How We Can All Help the Planet!" **www.youtube.com**.

[3]Stiteler, S., e-mail correspondence, October 23, 2008.

[4]Easterling, J., personal interview, March 29, 2009.

[5]Joseph, J.A., et al., "Age-Related Neurodegeneration and Oxidative Stress Putative Nutritional Intervention," *Neurologic Clinics*, vol. 16, no. 3 (1998): 747–55.

[6]Semba, R.D., and G. Dagnelie, "Are Lutein and Zeaxanthin Conditionally Essential Nutrients for Eye Health?" *Medical Hypotheses*, vol. 61, no. 4 (2003): 465–72.

[7]King, F., and R. Steiner, *Rudolf Steiner and Holistic Medicine*. York Beach, ME: Nicolas-Hays: 1987.

[8]Grossarth-Maticek, R., et al., "Use of Iscador, an Extract of European Mistletoe (Viscum Album), in Cancer Treatment: Prospective Nonrandomized and Randomized Matched-Pair Studies Nested within a Cohort Study," *Alternative Therapies in Health and Medicine*, vol. 7, no. 3 (2001): 57.

Chapter Six

[1]Math/Science Nucleus, "Importance of Water," **http://msnucleus.org/watersheds/General/importance.htm**.

[2]Uthman, E., e-mail correspondence, September 3, 2008.

[3]Teton, S., e-mail correspondence, May 23, 2009.

[4]Carroll, C., e-mail correspondence, April 3, 2009.

[5]Melson, E., personal interview, February 3, 2009.

[6]Schatz, A., *Teaching Science with Soil*. Emmaus, PA: Rodale, 1972.

[7]Becker, P., personal interview and e-mail communication, November 4, 2008.

[8]Ni, M., personal interview, March 14, 2009.

Chapter Seven

[1]Mangini, K., e-mail correspondence, April 18, 2009.

[2]Hill, N., *Think and Grow Rich*. Mineola, NY: Dover Publications, 2007.

[3]Miller, P., "Swarm Behavior," *National Geographic,* July 2007: **http://ngm.nationalgeographic.com/ngm/0707/feature5/text3.html**.

Chapter Eight

[1]Rouse, S., "Mystery of Ancient Astronomical Calculator Unveiled," *Innovations Report:* **www.innovations-report.com/html/reports/physics_astronomy/report-75167.html**.

[2]Tapia, P., "Stargazing Wines," *in,* June 2009: **www.in-lan.com/en/0906/feature.html**.

[3]Hallowell, E., "What's It Like to Have ADD?" *Bridges of Opportunity,* winter 2004.

[4]Worley, L., e-mail correspondence, January 26, 2009.

Chapter Nine

[1]"Carl Lewis: Beyond Sport Part 1," **www.youtube.com**.

[2]Lee, L., personal interview, February 16, 2009.

Chapter Ten

[1]Semprevivo, M., e-mail correspondence, January 22, 2008.

[2]Riou, P., "Fibonacci Number Sequence," **www.futures-investor.co.uk/fibonacci_number_sequence.htm**.

[3]Britton, J., "Fibonacci Numbers in Nature," **http://britton.disted.camosun.bc.ca/fibslide/jbfibslide.htm**.

[4]Garland, T., *Fascinating Fibonaccis: Mystery and Magic in Numbers.* Palo Alto, CA: Dale Seymour Publications, 1987.

[5]Meisner, G., "Fibonacci Spirals," **http://goldennumber.net**.

[6]Greer, J.M., *Techniques for Geometric Transformation.* St. Paul, MN: Llewellyn, 2002.

[7]Jean, R.V., *Phyllotaxis: A Systemic Study in Plant Morphogenesis.* New York: Cambridge University Press, 1994.

[8]Zaboski, D., phone interview, April 24, 2009.

[9]Ball, P., *The Self-Made Tapestry: Pattern Formation in Nature.* Oxford, England: Oxford University Press, 1999.

[10]James, R., "Your Gemologist," **www.yourgemologist.com**.

[11]Jhon, M.S., *The Water Puzzle and the Hexagonal Key.* 1st ed. Orem, UT: Uplifting Press, 2004.

[12]Easterling, J., personal interview, March 29, 2009.

[13]Wood, M., phone interview, April 6, 2008.

[14]Aguilar, J., e-mail correspondence, July 15, 2009.

Chapter Eleven

[1]Benyus, J. *Biomimicry.* New York: Quill, 1998.

[2]Trewavas, A.J., *Molecular and Cellular Aspects of Calcium in Plant Development* (Nato ASI Series, Series A, Life Sciences vol. 104). New York: Plenum Press, 1986.

[3]Jenks, T., phone interview, March 14, 2008.

[4]Welles, A., personal interview, May 3, 2009.

[5]Aguilar, J., e-mail correspondence, July 15, 2009.

[6]Cohen, J., e-mail correspondence, February 13, 2009.

[7]Seeberg, K., e-mail correspondence, March 17, 2009.

[8]Teton, S., e-mail correspondence, July 5, 2009.

Chapter Twelve

[1]Harper, S., "The Way of Wilderness," **www.stevenkharper.com/way ofwilderness.html**.

[2]Chester, T., "Mountain Lion Attacks on People in the U.S. and Canada," **http://tchester.org/sgm/lists/lion_attacks.html**.

Chapter Thirteen

[1]Etheridge, G., personal interview, September 23, 2008.

[2]Stolarczyk, J., e-mail correspondence, February 10, 2009.

[3]USDA Food Safety and Inspection Service, "Meat Packaging Materials," **www.fsis.usda.gov/Factsheets/Meat_Packaging_Materials/index.asp**.

[4]*Consumer Reports,* "Seeing Red: Spoiled Meat May Look Fresh," July 2006: **www.consumerreports.org/cro/consumer-protection/consumer-interest/meat-treated-with-carbon-monoxide-spoiled-meat-may-look-fresh-7-06/overview/0607_spoiled-meat_ov.htm**.

[5]LocalHarvest, "Community Supported Agriculture," **www.localharvest .org/csa**.

Chapter Fourteen

[1]Taubes, G., "Do We Really Know What Makes Us Healthy?" *The New York Times,* September 16, 2007.

[2]Jeanne Lenzer, "Wonder Drugs That Can Kill: Modern Pharmaceutical 'Breakthroughs' Sometimes Do More Harm than Good," *Discover,* July 2008: **http://discovermagazine.com/2008/jul/20-wonder-drugs-that-can-kill**.

[3]Critser, G., *Generation Rx: How Prescription Drugs Are Altering American Lives, Minds, and Bodies.* New York: Houghton Mifflin, 2005.

[4]Buhner, S.H., *The Lost Language of Plants: The Ecological Importance of Plant Medicines to Life on Earth.* White River Junction, VT: Chelsea Green, 2002.

[5]Schipper, J., e-mail correspondence, February 26, 2009.

Chapter Fifteen

[1]Garner, D., phone interview, October 25, 2008.

[2]Garcia, D., *The Future of Food,* 2007: **www.thefutureoffood.com/resources.htm**.

[3]Hauter, W., "Irradiation: Expensive, Ineffective, and Impractical," **www.foodandwaterwatch.org/food/foodirradiation/copy_of_food-irradiation**.

[4]Barnard, N., "Blame Industrial Animal Operations for Disease Outbreaks Among Humans," *AgWeek,* February 23, 2009: **www.agweek.com/articles/?id=2665&article_id=13678&property_id=41**.

[5]McAfee, M., phone interview, February 12, 2008.

[6]Buhner, S., *One Spirit Many Peoples: A Manifesto for Earth Spirituality.* Niwot, CO: Rinehart, 1997.

❧ ❧ ❧   ❧ ❧ ❧

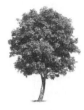

ACKNOWLEDGMENTS

With Immense Gratitude . . .

I read a story about a whale that was tangled up in rope at the shore. All the people of the town got together to cut the ropes and save its life. After all the ropes were cut and before the whale swam out to sea, it purposely looked into each person's eyes one by one, showing its immense gratitude. . . . So here's *my* opportunity to point out each of the people who supported me in writing this book so that it could be set free into the world.

Louise Hay is my fairy godmother who helped make this book a reality. Louise, you are a visionary and positive light on this planet. *Wow!*

A huge thank-you to Reid Tracy at Hay House who gave the go-ahead for this book. Reid, you rock! The Hay House team: the superb, gifted guidance of editors extraordinaire Jill Kramer and Lisa Mitchell. Lisa has been so instrumental in making this book the best it can be with her wise, kind, and insightful help. And thanks to Christy Salinas; Johanne Mahaffey; Bryn Best, for her beautiful and artistic creativity for the cover; and Julie Davison, for her wonderful book design.

The following book coaches, Adriane Smith, Katy Koontz, and Nancy Peske, sprinkled in their magic. All were wonderful delights and such a pleasure to work with. But mostly, I worked with my mom, editing together almost daily, discussing every idea, word choice, and comma possible more times than I can count.

These amazing people gave me feedback: Janet Baghoomian, Barbara Belt, Laurie Goldstein, Michele Martin, Michael Meissner, Dean Minerd, and George Sobol.

To my wonderful angels: Melvin Allen, Sherrie Allen, Elizabeth Amini, Kathy Angileri, Dave Arnoth, David Barrett, Lynne Barstow, Tina Bilezikjian, Connie Bishaf, Keith Bishaf, Jacqui Brandywine, Raie Mcphearson Bronze, Laura and Jim Cook, Bruce Dickson, Mia Earl, Leila Ferrer, Dr. Ai, Rick Frishman, Bill Gladstone, Laurie Goldstein, Harijiwan and Erin, Mary Hulnick, Ron Hulnick, Wendy Jackson, Cindy Jones, Jack Jones, Lisa Klinker, Henry Klinker, Chef Bob Knopik, Robert Kuang Ju Wu, Kay Larson, Linda Neiman Lee, Lee Levitt, Roxanna Lisenby, Diane Longbottom, Judy Loogee Logue Gibbons, Karen Mangini, Master Bob McCarthy, Sr., Nara-mae Munster, Vicki Nevarde, Sally Oster, Teddy (Axel) Osterloff, Chris Piccione-Politis, Marnie Pomerantz, Chris Seitz, Johnny Seitz, Karen Seeberg, Leslie Sloane, Mia, G.P., and Valentina Salardi, Chef Susan Teton, Sat Siri, Rebecc0a Underwood, Bijan and Noray Maaj, Jonathan and Melissa Maaj, Howard Wills, Cindy Wilkes, Kathryn Wilkes, Roy Wilkes, Len Worley, Robin Harlan-Zaboski, and Dave Zaboski. Thank you to the people at Woodland Hills library, especially Jennifer Christensen, Leslie Hayes, Stephanie Herman, Asif Khan, and Mike Syung.

And I have immense gratitude for my dad, Roy Wilkes, who taught me how to be creative, to ask, and to go for it.

But most of all, I have enormous heartfelt appreciation for my mom, who's my book buddy. She was instrumental and joyful in helping with every aspect of the book, from conception to completion. While on the phone, we went over and over the manuscript together while reading it from our computers, choosing the best thoughts and words, for more than a year and a half. My mom helped make writing the book a delight and a reality. Without her, it would have taken twice as long and been half as fun. How great is that!

🌿 🌿 🌿 🌿 🌿 🌿

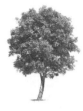

ABOUT THE AUTHOR

Elaine Wilkes, Ph.D., N.C., M.A., a self-proclaimed "learning addict," ultimately discovered that the answers to most of life's questions are revealed in Nature. (Just like Dorothy's ruby slippers, the solutions she sought were there the whole time—in plain sight right outside her front door!)

Elaine has a Ph.D. in alternative medicine/naturopathy, a master's degree in psychology, and degrees in nutrition and communications. She weaves together herbalism; Chinese and Ayurvedic medicine; and Christian, Taoist, Native American, and shamanic wisdom and combines them with science and intuition to ingeniously unravel Nature's secret messages.

Elaine skillfully merges her acting background (she has appeared in numerous television shows and movies, and in more than 75 TV commercials) with her vast research and imaginative insights into Nature to give memorable, thought-provoking presentations. Her enthusiasm and high energy are infectious and refreshing.

As a LEED™ (Leadership in Energy and Environmental Design) accredited professional, Elaine teaches easy ways to "go green" and shows individuals and businesses how to cut costs by becoming more environmentally friendly. Find out how Elaine can help you, your group, or your business save money and the planet by visiting her Website: **www.ElaineWilkes.com.**

🍃 🍃 🍃   🍃 🍃 🍃

We hope you enjoyed this Hay House book.
If you'd like to receive our online catalog featuring additional
information on Hay House books and products, or if you'd like
to find out more about the Hay Foundation, please contact:

Hay House, Inc.
P.O. Box 5100
Carlsbad, CA 92018-5100

(760) 431-7695 or **(800) 654-5126**
(760) 431-6948 (fax) or **(800) 650-5115 (fax)**
www.hayhouse.com® • **www.hayfoundation.org**

Published and distributed in Australia by:
Hay House Australia Pty. Ltd., 18/36 Ralph St., Alexandria NSW 2015
Phone: 612-9669-4299 • *Fax:* 612-9669-4144 • www.hayhouse.com.au

Published and distributed in the United Kingdom by:
Hay House UK, Ltd., 292B Kensal Rd., London W10 5BE
Phone: 44-20-8962-1230 • *Fax:* 44-20-8962-1239 • www.hayhouse.co.uk

Published and distributed in the Republic of South Africa by:
Hay House SA (Pty), Ltd., P.O. Box 990, Witkoppen 2068 • *Phone/Fax:*
27-11-467-8904 • info@hayhouse.co.za • www.hayhouse.co.za

Published in India by:
Hay House Publishers India, Muskaan Complex, Plot No. 3, B-2,
Vasant Kunj, New Delhi 110 070 • *Phone:* 91-11-4176-1620
Fax: 91-11-4176-1630 • www.hayhouse.co.in

Distributed in Canada by:
Raincoast, 9050 Shaughnessy St., Vancouver, B.C. V6P 6E5
Phone: (604) 323-7100 • *Fax:* (604) 323-2600 • www.raincoast.com

Take Your Soul on a Vacation

Visit **www.HealYourLife.com®** to regroup, recharge, and reconnect
with your own magnificence. Featuring blogs, mind-body-spirit news,
and life-changing wisdom from Louise Hay and friends.

Visit **www.HealYourLife.com** today!

HEAL YOUR LIFE ♥

Take Your Soul on a Vacation

Get your daily dose of inspiration today at **www.HealYourLife.com®**. Brimming with all of the necessary elements to ease your mind and educate your soul, this Website will become the foundation from which you'll start each day. This essential site delivers the latest in mind, body, and spirit news and real-time content from your favorite Hay House authors.

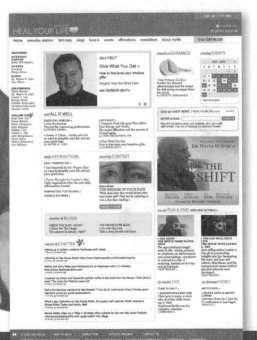

Make It Your Home Page Today!

www.HealYourLife.com®